Dental Implants for Hygienists and Therapists

Dental Implants for Hygienists and Therapists

Ulpee Darbar BDS, MSc, FDS(Rest Dent)RCS, FHEA

Consultant in Restorative Dentistry
Eastman Dental Hospital
London, UK

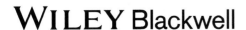

This edition first published 2022
© 2022 John Wiley and Sons Ltd

The right of Ulpee Darbar to be identified as the author of this work has been asserted in accordance with law.

Registered Offices
John Wiley & Sons, Inc., 111 River Street, Hoboken, NJ 07030, USA
John Wiley & Sons Ltd, The Atrium, Southern Gate, Chichester, West Sussex, PO19 8SQ, UK

Editorial Office
9600 Garsington Road, Oxford, OX4 2DQ, UK

For details of our global editorial offices, customer services, and more information about Wiley products visit us at www.wiley.com.

Wiley also publishes its books in a variety of electronic formats and by print-on-demand. Some content that appears in standard print versions of this book may not be available in other formats.

The work presented has been either been undertaken directly by the editor or the editor has been involved in overseeing the work.

Library of Congress Cataloging-in-Publication Data
Names: Darbar, Ulpee R., author.
Title: Dental implants for hygienists and therapists / Ulpee Darbar, Eastman Dental Hospital, London, UK.
Description: Hoboken, NJ : John Wiley & Sons, 2022. | Includes bibliographical references and index.
Identifiers: LCCN 2021053096 (print) | LCCN 2021053097 (ebook) | ISBN 9781119763826 (paperback) | ISBN 9781119763833 (pdf) | ISBN 9781119763840 (epub)
Subjects: LCSH: Dental implants. | Teeth--Transplantation.
Classification: LCC RK667.I45 D37 2022 (print) | LCC RK667.I45 (ebook) | DDC 617.6/93--dc23/eng/20211220
LC record available at https://lccn.loc.gov/2021053096
LC ebook record available at https://lccn.loc.gov/2021053097

Cover image: Courtesy of Ulpee Darbar
Cover design by Wiley

Set in 9.5/12.5pt STIXTwoText by Integra Software Services Pvt. Ltd, Pondicherry, India

C9781119763826_280322

Printed and bound by CPI Group (UK) Ltd, Croydon, CR0 4YY

Contents

Glossary

Abutment: The component of an implant that interfaces with the implant fixture and the prosthetic entity. Retained with a screw or can be adapted for a prosthesis to be cemented. Made of titanium, alloyed metals, gold; zirconia; ceramic. They can be preformed and come as straight or angled or custom made.

Analogue: Replica of the implant fixture or the abutment which is used by the laboratory to make the prosthesis.

Abutment driver: Instrument used to connect the abutment to the fixture.

Abutment healing cap: A temporary cover used to protect the implant fixture head during the healing period.

Abutment–implant interface: The surface of contact between the implant fixture and the abutment.

Abutment-level impression: Impression of the abutment taken once the abutment is connected to the implant fixture either directly through conventional impressions or indirectly through an impression coping.

Abutment Screw: The screw used to connect the abutment to the implant fixture and has different features depending if it is a single crown or a bridge. It is torqued to the final position.

Allogenic bone: Bone from the same species.

Alloplastic material: Material of synthetic origin that does not have human or animal origin.

Anti-rotation: A feature that prevents rotational movement

Barrier membrane: A material used to exclude cells from invading into the defect allowing the preferred cells to grow into the defect. When used technique is called guided bone or tissue regeneration. Membrane can be resorbable or non-resorbable. Made of collagen or synthetic derivatives which are resorbable or titanium or polytetrafluorethylene (PTFE) which are non resorbable.

Bicortical stabilisation: Used when both the superior and inferior cortices of bone are used to obtain stability of the implant.

Bisphosphonate-related osteonecrosis of the jaw (BRONJ): Also called medication-related necrosis, it is the necrosis of bone related to bisphosphonates.

Bone to implant contact: A term used to describe the direct contact of bone to the implant.

Bone to implant interface: The line of separation between the living bone and implant fixture surface.

CAD-CAM: Computer-aided design computer-aided manufacture used to plan, design and construct implant restorations. It forms part of the digital workflow.

Connective tissue attachment: The mechanism by which the connective tissue attaches to the implant.

Countersinking: Bone preparation of the crestal aspect using special drivers to allow subcrestal (below the bone) placement of the implant shoulder.

Cover screw: Fits over the implant head to protect it when the gum tissue is closed over it and the fixture is submerged.

Dental implant: A screw made of titanium that is screwed into the jawbone using specialised and specified techniques to resemble a tooth root.

Diagnostic wax up: Procedure in which the teeth are created to match the planned restoration and used in planning and also for construction of a radiographic and surgical guide.

Digital workflow: A workflow that uses digital technology to convert analogue structures into a digital format.

External connection: The connection that protrudes on top of the implant fixture platform and connects the prosthesis to the fixture.

Fixed prosthesis: A prosthesis that is fixed to the implant fixture which the patient cannot remove for cleaning.

Fixation screws and tacks: Used to stabilise membranes or block grafts to the underlying bone.

Fixture: Endosteal dental implant.

Guide drill: The first drill used to open the cortical bone at the implant site during implant surgery.

Guided bone regeneration: Technique used to selectively allow bone cells to populate the defect.

Healing abutment/cap: Used after the first- or second-stage surgery to connect the implant fixture to the oral cavity.

Implant stability: Clinical evaluation of the implant assessing its degree of stability.

Implant substructure: The metal framework onto which the crown or prosthesis is connected.

Impression coping: A device used to register the position of the dental implant or abutment.

Immediate loading: The prosthesis is placed underload at the same time as implant fixture placement.

Internal connection: The connection which sits inside the body of the implant fixture and links the implant fixture to the prosthesis. It comes in different configurations.

Peri-implant diseases: Include peri-implant mucositis where there is reversible inflammation of the gingival tissues and peri-implantitis where there is irreversible loss of bone with inflammation.

Prosthetic screw: Screw used to connect the prosthesis to the abutment.

Primary stability: Mechanical stability achieved when the implant fixture is placed. Also knows as the initial stability.

Provisional restoration: Temporary restoration placed whilst the tissues are healing.

Radiographic marker: A radio-opaque material incorporated into the radiographic guide to show the position.

Radiographic stent/guide: Used to direct the position of the tooth in relation to the underlying bone. Worn by the patient when having the radiograph or CT scan.

Regeneration: Technique used to reconstitute tissues lost through disease.

Surgical guide/template: Used during the surgical implant placement to guide the placement of the implant fixture to be placed in the correct restoratively driven position and angulation.

Torque driver: Instrument used to apply the correct level of tightening force (torque) to the screws.

Two-stage surgery: When the implant fixture is covered over by the soft tissue and a minor procedure is undertaken to uncover the fixture.

1

History of Dental Implants

The concept of dental implants dates as far back as 2000 BC when carved bamboo pegs were originally used to replace missing teeth. A dental implant is a prosthetic device made of alloplastic material implanted either into the oral tissues beneath the mucosal and/or the periosteal layer and/or within the bone to provide retention and support for a fixed or removable prosthesis. When inserted into the bone, the implants are called endo-osseous implants.

Around 3000 years ago, Egyptians used metal pegs to replace teeth, and it was not until the 1930s the concept of modern implantology came into existence with progressive development of methods used to replace missing teeth (Table 1.1). The materials from which dental implants are made should be biocompatible, corrosion resistant, and encourage bone ingrowth and biofunctionality.

During 1939–60s the concept of the 'in the bone' (endosteal) implant arose with the first cylindrical endo-osseous solid screw implant with threads both internally and externally with a smooth gingival collar and healing cap being placed. Following this during the 1940s, a spiral stainless steel post type endosseous implant with a design that allowed bone to grow into the implant emerged and Dahl in Germany, around the same time, introduced the concept of the subperiosteal implant with mucosal inserts (Figure 1.1). This implant was made of cobalt-chromium molybedenum with a direct impression of the struts on the ridge crest taken to construct the denture. Throughout the 1940s–50s variations on the original Dahl design emerged in an attempt to make the provision of implants simpler and included the use of vitallium implants in 1948, the Linkow endo-osseous blade vent implant in 1966 with different designs for the maxilla and mandible (Figure 1.2), the ramus frame implant in 1970, made of stainless steel (Figure 1.3) and mandibular transosseal implant which engaged the lower border of the mandible with inserts projecting into the mouth to support a prosthesis (Figure 1.4). The ramus frame and tranossteal implants were predominantly designed for patients with atrophic mandibles who had difficulties wearing dentures and were used to aide denture retention to improve function.

The key challenge with these older implant systems was biocompatibility, the lack of fusion to the jawbone resulting in recurring infections after a period of time and the complex surgical techniques needed to insert the implants leading to limited use aimed at

Dental Implants for Hygienists and Therapists, First Edition. Ulpee Darbar.
© 2022 John Wiley & Sons Ltd. Published 2022 by John Wiley & Sons Ltd.

Table 1.1 Progressive Development of Methods used for Tooth Replacement.

500–2500 BC	300–600 AD	800 AD	1500–1800s	1809	1913
– Egyptians tried splinting teeth using gold ligature wires – Eustracians used customised soldered gold bands from animals and oxen bone	– Phoenicians used Ivory to carve teeth used as bridge replacements – Mayans introduced the concept of implants when they tried to use 'Pieces of Shells' as implants to replace mandibular teeth; Radiographs taken in the 1970s of such mandibles show compact bone formation around the implants (bone similar to that around blade implants)	Hondurans used a stone implant and placed this in the mandible	Europeans used cadaver teeth for allotrans-plantation	J Maggiolo inserted a gold implant tube into a fresh extraction socket and after healing a crown was added; other materials used were silver capsules, corrugated porcelain	Dr Greenfield placed a '24-gauge hollow latticed cylinder of iridio-platinum soldered with 24-karat gold' as an artificial root to 'fit exactly the circular incision made for it in the jawbone of the patient'

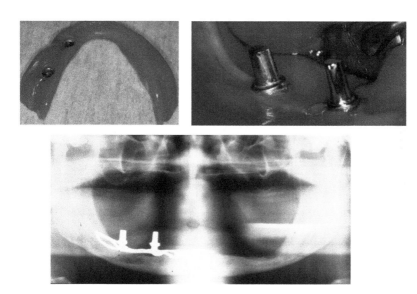

Figure 1.1 Subperiosteal implants in the mouth.

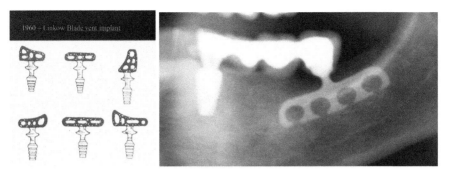

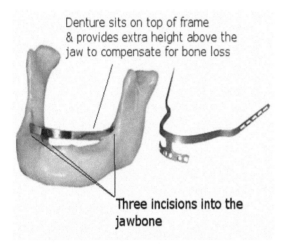

Figure 1.2   Blade vent implants.

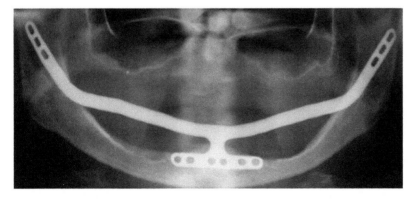

Figure 1.3   Ramus implants.

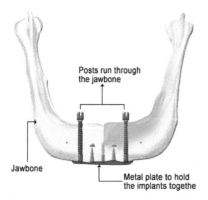

Posts run through
the jawbone

Jawbone

Metal plate to hold
the implants togethe

Figure 1.4   Mandibular tranossteal implant.

specific patient groups. Additionally, the infections led to secondary issues with bone resorption compounding the existing issues.

In the 1950s, an orthopaedic surgeon, Per Ingvar Branemark, accidentally found, during the study of bone healing and regeneration, that a titanium cylinder fused together with the bone in the femur of a rabbit. He hypothesised that this fusion could be utilised in field of dental implants and placed the first dental implant made of commercially pure titanium in a human volunteer in 1965. This finding introduced the concept of osseointegration which forms the basis of today's endo-osseous dental implants. Osseointegration became accepted as a worldwide phenomenon when the concept was launched at the Toronto World Conference in 1982. At around the same time, whilst Branemark was looking at a two-stage threaded implant, Schroeder and his group were independently evaluating the use of a one-piece root form implant made with a hollow design and a roughened surface (Figure 1.5a, b).

Since the introduction of osseointegration, in the late 1980s, as a predictable method of tooth replacement, growing confidence and predictability has led to the widespread use of dental implants moving from edentulism to partial edentulism including single teeth and those with extensive tissue and tooth loss usually seen in patients who have suffered traumatic injuries and congenital anomalies (e.g. Hypodontia). This progressive change has led to the focus changing from improving function to include aesthetics and psychological well-being alongside the need to address patient expectations.

Dental implantology continues to evolve with concomitant modification of implant screw designs, surfaces and techniques used for implant placement and restoration aimed at reducing integration healing times, optimising function and aesthetics alongside predictability. These changes have led to newer concepts for tooth replacement being considered which include the use of zygomatic implants in those with atrophic maxillae, the mini implants and the 'All-on-Four' concept whereby the teeth are extracted and implants placed and restored all on the same day. Additionally, the advent

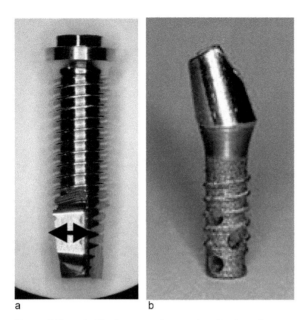

a   b

Figure 1.5   a, b: The Branemark two-piece implant fixture and the Shroeder one-piece hollow cylinder implant.

of digital technology has enabled clinicians and technicians to push this clinical envelop even further with digital systems being used for planning, surgical placement and restoration without any analogue interfaces being used. Whilst, we live in a fast-moving world driven by technology and systems geared to meet patient demands, the biological envelop in which we as clinicians have to work has seen little change and as clinicians we need to be cognizant of this challenge commonly referred to as 'patient and site' related factors.

Today there are in excess of 250 implant systems on the market with varying design features, many of which resemble either one or more features of the eight mainstream implant systems. Table 1.2 shows the development of different key implant systems since 1982.

Key Learning Points

- Be able to describe the older systems, as patients may attend for treatment with these systems
- Being able to recognise the older systems to assist with management
- Be able to explain to patients possible problems and issues with infections
- Be aware of challenges associated with evolution of the concept of dental implants

Table 1.2 Some of the Mainstream Dental Implant Systems.

1977	Branemark Implants
1982	Launch of Osseointegration
1982	Non-submerged implant system: ITI Corevent implant system
1985	Biocon
1987	IMZ
1989	3i
1990	Astra
1999	Straumann Synocta
Late 1990s	Frident (Frialit 2, Xive)
Early 2000	Ankylos and similar
Mid-2000 onwards	Modification of the earlier implant systems with newer surfaces, shapes and designs

References

1 Abraham, C. (2014). A brief historical perspectice on dental implants, their surface coatings and their treatments. *Open Dentistry Journal* 8: 50–55.

2 Branemark, P.I. and Zarb, G. (1985). *Tissue Integrated Prosthesis: Osseointegration in Clinical Dentistry*. Quintessence Publishing.

3 Rajput, R., Chouhan, Z., Sindhu, M., Sundararajan, S., and Chouhan, R. (2016). A brief chronological review of dental implant history. *International Dental Journal of Student's Research* 4 (3): 105–107.

2

Osseointegration

Osseointegration (OI) was first defined at the light microscopic level as a 'direct structural and functional connection between ordered living bone and the surface of a load carrying implant' (Branemark 1983). The phenomenon involves a complex interaction between the implant, bone and tissue interface (Figure 2.1). The process involves two stages with an initial biomechanical interlocking between the implant body and alveolar bone, called primary stability, followed by the second stage which involves the biological fixation of the implant through bone remodelling and apposition, called secondary stability, with each stage being influenced by various factors and steps being followed during the placement of the implant (Figure 2.2). Primary implant stability plays an essential role in successful osseointegration and is dependent on the implant geometry, the bone quality and quantity as well as the site preparation technique.

Concept

The original concept of OI was redefined at the clinical level by Zarb and Albrektsson (1983) as a 'time dependent healing process whereby clinically asymptomatic rigid fixation of alloplastic materials is achieved and maintained in bone during functional loading'. The histologic appearance resembled a functional ankylosis with no intervening fibrous or connective tissue between bone and implant surface (Figure 2.3). The first implants, known as 'Branemark Implants', were made of pure machined titanium surfaces and had to be covered over by the gum flap after surgical placement for at least six months to allow the screw to integrate into the jaw bone. Today with an improved understanding of the concept and changes in implant screw designs and surface modifications, the healing times have reduced with implants being restored at the same time as placement with healing periods of 0–8 weeks. Figure 2.4 shows the different healing time lines for dental implants and their restorations. The original clinical definition of osseointegration thus needs updating with removal of the word 'time dependent' as a fixed period of healing before loading is no longer an absolute requirement.

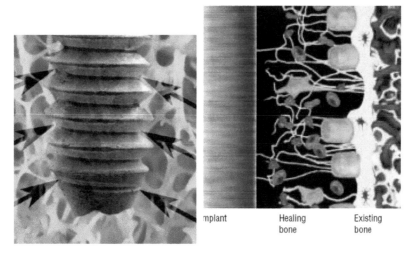

Figure 2.1 Bone to implant contact in osseointegration.

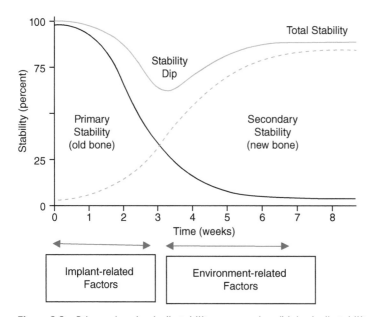

Figure 2.2 Primary (mechanical) stability vs secondary (biological) stability.

Factors Affecting Osseointegration

Factors affecting osseointegration can be divided into implant related and environment related (Table 2.1).

• Implant-related factors:

These factors primarily affect the mechanical interlocking of the implant and are thus fundamental to facilitating OI. They include the material of which the implant is made (biocompatibility), the design features of the implant and the macroscopic and

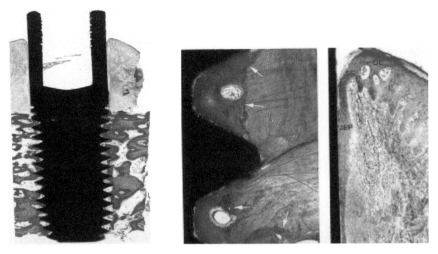

Figure 2.3 Osseointegration showing the close interface of the implant surface to bone with no intervening soft tissue.

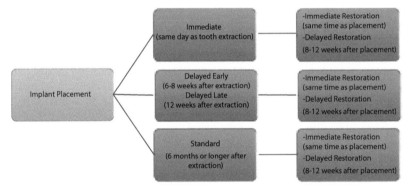

Figure 2.4 Healing time lines for implant placement and restoration.

microscopic surface features of the implant. Progressive changes in these features have enabled reduced healing periods as a result of the improved primary stability at the time of implant placement.

- Implant Materials
  The material of which the implant is made does not directly influence the mechanical stability of the implant but ensures biocompatibility.

- Commercially pure titanium (cpTI):
  This material has excellent biocompatibility, and its bioactivity is related to the immediate formation of a stable and inert oxide layer on its outer surface when exposed to air. It is classified into grades 1–4 depending on the purity and processing oxygen content with Grade 1 being the most pure with the lowest oxygen content (0.18%) and Grade 4 being the least pure with the highest oxygen content (0.4%). The different grades contain varying amounts of contaminants such as iron for corrosion

Table 2.1 Factors Affecting Osseointegration.

Implant-Related **Mechanical Stability = Primary Stability** **(Initial Period)**	Environment (Host)-Related **Biological Stability = Secondary Stability**
Materials (Biocompatiblity) ● Commercially pure titanium ● Titanium alloys ● Zirconium	*Status of the Host Bed* ● Vascularity ● Quality of bone : Type I, II, III, IV
Design ● Shape ● Threads	*Surgical Site Preparation* ● No overheating ● Ample cooling ● Technique ● Sequential drilling
Surface ● Machined (turned) ● Plasma sprayed/laser ● Sandblasted ● Acid etched ● Anodised ● Coated ● Chemically treated	*Healing Periods* ● Influenced by above and need for augmentation ● Post-operative trauma ● Smoking ● Aftercare ● Prosthesis
Diameter and Length ● Narrow, regular, wide ● Short, standard, long	*Loading Conditions* ● Immediate ● Early ● Delayed ● Standard
Influenced by Operator Related Knowledge, Skill and Competence	

resistance, aluminium for increased strength and reduced density and vanadium which scavenges the aluminium thus imparting corrosion resistance. Grade 4 cpTI has the highest strength, highest passivity and a modulus of elasticity comparable to bone and is therefore the material of choice for manufacturing dental implants. Its key disadvantages are the low wear resistance and grey metal shine through in patients with thin gingival tissues contributing to compromised aesthetics.

- Titanium alloys:
  The alloying of cpTI enhances the strength and wear resistance of the material.

- Titanium, Aluminium and Vanadium Alloy (Ti6Al4V):
  This alloy is mainly used for dental implants and contains 6% aluminium, 4% vanadium, up to 0.25% iron and 0.2% oxygen with the rest being titanium. The material has excellent fatigue properties and corrosion resistance with a low elastic modulus leading to a 'stress shielding' effect due to the mismatch between the implant material and surrounding

bone. The alloy releases small amounts of aluminium and vanadium ions and can be associated with allergic reactions, cytotoxic effects and neurological disorders. Implant systems made of titanium alloys usually tend to be slightly cheaper than those using cpTI.

- Titanium-Zirconium Alloy (Ti-Zr):
  This alloy has been shown to be biocompatible, bioactive and mechanically stable and has comparable properties to cpTi with a reported tendency to significantly improve osteoblast adhesion to the implant surface. The 'Roxolid' implants manufactured by the Straumann Company are made of this alloy and have been used for more than five years with good success rates. The strength of the material enables smaller implant diameters to be made with internal connections.

- Zirconium/Ceramic
  Zirconium, a ceramic biocompatible biomaterial, has gained popularity as an implant material due to its aesthetics and was first tested during the 1990s as an implant material. The oxide form of zirconium has the capacity to create OI of a lesser quality and etching techniques have been used to improve the quality and extent of the OI. There are two zirconium implants available on the market. The 'Ceraroot' implant is an acid-etched zirconium implant (Oral Iceberg) and Straumann Pure ZLA is also an acid-etched ceramic implant (Figure 2.5a, 2.5b).

- Implant Design
  The design of an implant facilitates the primary stability during the placement of the implant and includes the shape and thread configuration of the implant. Other parameters such as diameter and length are also important and influence primary stability indirectly.

  - Implant shape
    The implant shape ensures there is a good approximation between the bone and implant and facilitates force distribution to the bone. Three shapes, cylindrical, parallel sided and tapered, have been used with the cylindrical form implants manufactured as unthreaded implants inserted using a 'press-fit' action into the prepared site (Figure 2.6). These implants are no longer available due to compromised treatment outcomes. Parallel-sided and tapered/conical screw (also called threaded) form implants have been used with the former being more popular until recently where hybrid designs combining the features of both these shapes becoming more widely used (Figure 2.7). These hybrid implants are designed to increase the contact area between the implant and bone as well as relieving stress concentrations due to the different thread designs thereby improving the stability enabling reduced healing times (Figure 2.8). Most implant systems have introduced these 'hybrid' versions into their portfolio whilst still retaining the standard implant designs.

- Implant threads
  The threads on a implant screw determine the degree to which the stability of the implant when placed is achieved and also facilitates the stress distribution to the bone. The degree of the stability achieved will be dependent on the profile and configuration of the threads called the thread depth and pitch (Figure 2.9). Screw form implants have threads that are

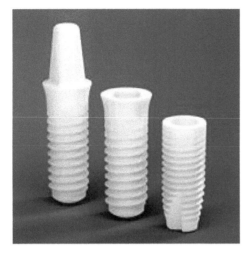

(a)

(b)

Figure 2.5   a. b: Zirconium implants. a: Straumann. b: Ceraroot.

designed to engage into the alveolar bone thereby improving primary stability and the sharper the thread pitch the better the stability. This is a feature that has been introduced into most implants systems as the surgical provision of implants has moved towards immediate and delayed placement. Figure 2.10 shows the different thread configurations and shapes which influence the stress concentration on the bone. Most implant systems adopt a combination of thread designs incorporating microthreads coronally with a tapering thread profile, double and triple thread configurations and increased thread width, pitch and depth. The use of microthreads coronally is deemed to increase the contact between the coronal bone and implant thus reducing the risk of coronal bone loss whereas, changes in thread pitch and depth are aimed at providing faster penetration into the bone thereby reducing risk of trauma to the bone. These changes in design have enabled improved primary stability thus contributing to faster osseointegration and healing (Figure 2.11a, 2.11b).

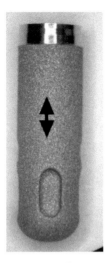

Figure 2.6 Cylindrical implants used with a press fit action for placement (IMZ implant with TPS-coated surface).

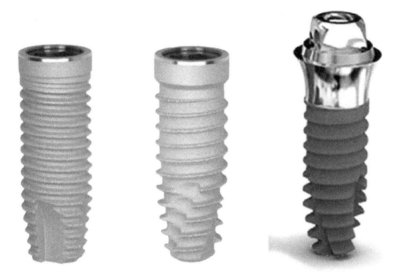

Figure 2.7 Parallel-sided and tapered implants.

- Implant Surfaces

  Surface topography of the implant influences the attraction of the osteoblasts to the implant surface with rough surfaces promoting osteogenesis by increasing the surface area over which the osteogenic cells can adhere and cellular activity takes place. The surface roughness can be described at the macroscopic (few mm to microns), microscopic (1–10microns) and nanometric (1–100 nm) level with the different levels having a profound effect on cellular healing accelerating the migration and proliferation of osteoblasts thereby improving the rate of osseointegration. Machined surface implants also

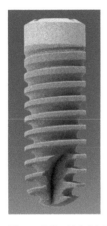

Figure 2.8   Hybrid-designed implant (parallel sided at the top; tapered apically).

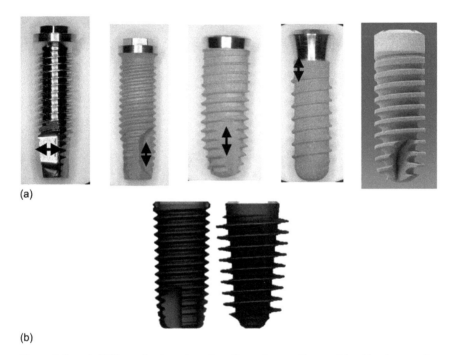

(a)

(b)

Figure 2.9   a, b: Different implant thread configurations. a: The machined implant on the right was the first implant and the change in the shape and design as well as the thread pitch is evident as you go from left to right. b: Different thread shapes and pitch (macrodesign).

known as 'turned' surfaces were the first to be used and whilst at a macroscopic level, the surface looked smooth, under the microscope the processing of the implants still created some irregularities on the surface. The irregularities increase the surface area and different techniques have been used with these implants being largely superseded by implants with different surface topographies. The two main methods used to modify the implant surface are either by removing material on the surface or adding material on the surface. The former include acid etching, blasting with an abrasive material and treatment with

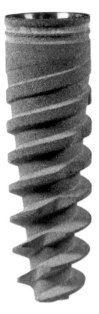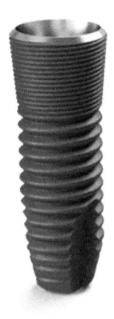

Figure 2.10 Shows the progressive change in an implant thread design: The implant on the left shows the change in the depth and pitch of the threads, and the implant on the right shows the microthreads at the top aimed at improving the contact with the coronal bone.

lasers whereas the latter includes hydroxyapatite coating and titanium plasma spraying, oxidation or anodization and deposition of nanoparticles by physical or chemical methods. Figure 2.12 shows the different surface topography and modifications associated with these methods. Plasma spraying and laser treatments are no longer used as the rate of integration was similar to that of the machined surfaces; however, laser treatment to promote gingival tissue adhesion, called the 'laser lock' has been used as a feature in one of the implant systems who state that this locking mechanism leads to an integration of the gingival tissue fibres to the surface. Table 2.2 shows the different generation of dental implants categorised according to the surface roughness.

- Implant Diameter and Length
  Implant diameters have changed over the years to enable improved profiles of the restorations. Early dental implants were available in one diameter (3.75 mm); however, as different types of teeth started being replaced with implants, the need for different diameters became evident to avoid 'mushroom' designs of the prosthesis. Implant diameters, today, fall into three groups, narrow (2.8–3.4 mm diameter), regular (3.75–4.1 mm) and wide (5.00–6 mm) with each group matching the type of tooth being replaced thus enabling the appropriate emergence profile of the restoration to maintain gingival tissue health (Figure 2.10) with each diameter group being colour coded enabling the correct components to be used. Implant lengths of up to 20 mm were advocated to achieve bicortical stabilisation where the border of the jaw bone and the alveolar crest was engaged to obtain stability. This concept has now evolved with the modified implant surfaces promoting healing with the average implant length being 11–13 mm. Whilst

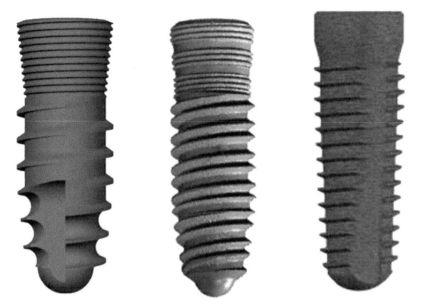

Figure 2.11a   The progressive change in the implant shape and thread profiles.

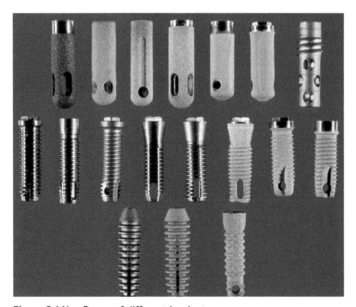

Figure 2.11b   Range of different implants.

previously, the shortest implant fixture advised was 7 mm, today the use of even shorter implant fixtures with lengths of 4–6 mm have become available as sites with compromised bone height are being considered for implant placement thus avoiding the need for advanced surgical interventions (Figure 2.13a, b). The use of the different diameters and lengths should be based on the outcome of the treatment plan agreed and finalised with the patient.

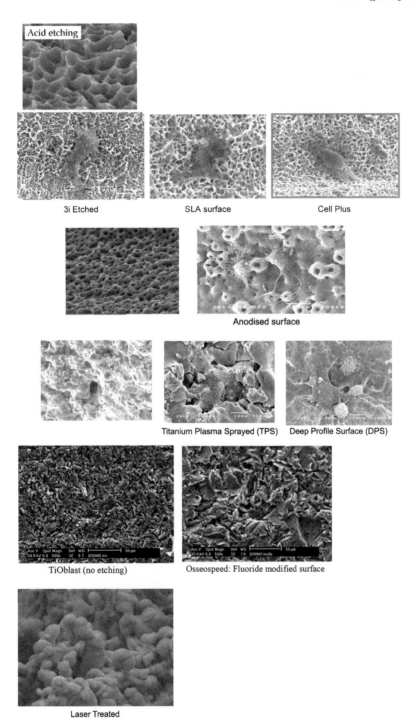

Figure 2.12 Electron Micrographs of the different surface topographies; acid etch, grit blasted, grit blasted and acid etched, anodised, plasma sprayed and laser treated. The SLA surface if both acid etched and grit blasted.

Table 2.2 Different Generations of Implant Systems with the Surface Modifications.

Generation	Surface Treatment	Type of System	Implant System
First	None	Blades, subperiosteal, ramus, transosteal	
Second	Weak	Machined (turned)	Old Branemark (Nobelbiocare);
		Titanium plasma sprayed (TPS)	Old Straumann
		Coated	Old IMZ
Third	Strong response	Moderately roughened surfaces	
		Sandblasted and etched	Straumann SLA Dentsply Frialit and Friadent
		Etched	Biomet 3i
		Anodised	Nobelbiocare TiUnite
		Blasted	Dentsply Astra TioBlast
		Laser ablation	Biohorizons Laser Lok
Fourth	Optimal response	Chemically active	Straumann SLA Active
		Fluoride coated	Dentsply Astra
		Calcium phosphate coating	Biomet 3i
		Bioactive glasses and bisphosphonates	Experimental

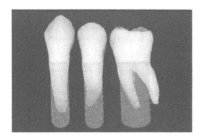
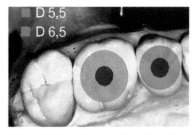
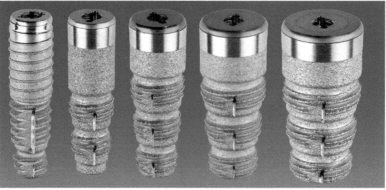

Figure 2.13a Implant diameters to match the type of tooth being replaced giving a better emergence profile for the restoration.

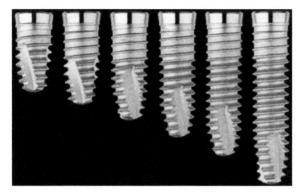

Figure 2.13b Different implant lengths.

● Environment-Related Factors

These factors influence the second phase of the osseointegration process during which the secondary stability of the implant is achieved. They include the status of the host bed, the surgical technique, healing period and loading conditions which determine the vascularity and the stability of the blood clot during the initial healing phase.

− Status of the host bed

The host bed is the alveolar bone and the surrounding soft tissues into which the implant is placed. The health of these tissues is crucial in determining how well the implant will integrate into the bone. Once the implant is placed, good vascularity (bleeding into the site) is needed to facilitate blood clot formation and remodelling of the cells into bone forming cells. In sites where the blood supply is compromised or reduced, the rate of osseointegration will be compromised due to the lack of bone-forming cells. The vascularity of the bone is dependent on the bone quality which is assessed by the ratio of the cortical to the cancellous bone and is described as Type 1, which is dense with little cancellous bone and Type IV which is soft with predominantly cancellous bone (Figure 2.14). Type 1 bone has poor vascularity due to the reduced number of bone cells and specialised techniques using a 'screw tap' are needed during the site preparation to minimise the risk of bone necrosis caused by pressure and overheating during placement. Type 4 bone is like 'quick sand' and has good vascularity but poor density and thus modifications, such as using specialised tools, e.g. bone condensers, during site preparation are needed to ensure that primary stability of the implant is achieved. Any movement of the implant or the blood clot during the initial healing period will lead to fibrous tissue formation and loss of osseointegration. Smoking affects the vascularity of the soft tissues and the bone and thus has a negative outcome on healing and therefore the quality of osseointegration but has also been associated with a higher risk of complications.

● Surgical Technique

The surgical technique is of paramount importance in determining predictability of osseointegration ensuring that the site is not overheated to more that 47°C during site preparation. This is achieved by the use of sharp drills, used sequentially at recommended speeds ranging from 800rpm to 1200 rpm depending on the implant system

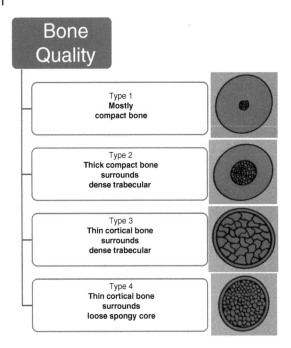

Figure 2.14 The different types of bone quality described by the ratio of the cortical to cancellous bone.

used. Throughout the drilling must be controlled with copious water cooling and minimal pressure to enable atraumatic site preparation. The cortical plate is usually perforated using a small round bur or sharp drill followed by gradually increasing diameter twist drills preparing the site to the required implant depth and diameter. The final drill is usually slightly smaller than the implant diameter which helps ensure good approximation of the implant surface to the bone (Figure 2.15). Parallel-sided implant placement advocates an intermittent drilling action, whereas the tapered or Hybrid designs, have matching drills that need to be used with a slight modification. Overprepared sites will either compromise the stability of the implant or cause trauma to the bone leading to failure of integration.

● Healing period
The healing periods with the early implants were crucial and could range upto six months; however, today with the newer generation implants, healing periods have reduced with implants being placed and restored on the same day. However, in all cases, treatment planning of the case is critical to the successful outcome of the implant placement and treatment and cases where extensive augmentation has been undertaken may still need 6–8 months for healing.

● Loading conditions
The loading of implants was restricted to six months with the early machined implants; however, loading protocols today have changed with immediate loading and loading within six weeks of placement being frequently applied. The time at which the implant

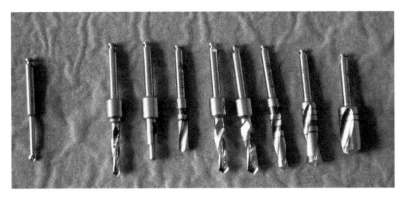

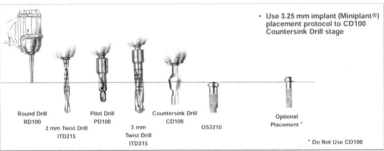

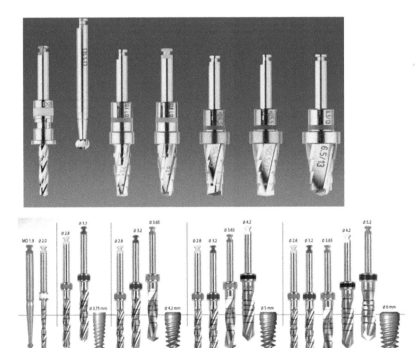

Figure 2.15 a, b, c: Drill sequence showing the incremental change in drill shape. a shows the parallel-sided drills with the line diagram; b shows the drills for a tapered implant and c shows the drill sizes alongside the implant diameters.

can be loaded will be determined by the quality of the bone and the primary stability obtained as well as the extent of augmentation undertaken at the time of implant placement. Loading protocols today are determined by the factors outlined above, but still remain crucial in the initial healing period. Inappropriate loading at the incorrect time will affect the quality of the integration leading to implant failure despite the newer designs promoting excellent primary stability due to the aggressive thread designs. Thus the type of loading protocol to be used should be considered at the outset during the planning stage and balanced against what is realistically possible.

Success Vs Survival

Implant treatment is influenced by a number of parameters. Success and survival are often used interchangeably to describe the outcomes of such treatment despite each term having a different meaning. A successful implant is one that is in situ and has not suffered any complications. It should, ideally, have been in function for at least five years with no history of either biological or mechanical complications and the surrounding tissues have remained healthy with stable marginal bone levels. Successfully placed implants will undergo 1.5 mm marginal bone resorption after placement during the first year of function followed by 0.1 mm annually thereafter depending on the type of placement and the technique used at placement. The bone remodelling around one piece implants (tissue level) is slightly lesser in the first two years with the annual remodelling being 0.1 mm as with the two-piece implant (bone level) systems. Marginal bone loss is one of the main criteria used to define success of dental implants. The criteria initially proposed by Albrektsson et al. (1986) are shown in Table 2.3a, and since this time others have included bleeding and peri-implant tissue health. Based on these criteria, success rates ranging from 90% to 95% over 10 years have been reported. To describe success, the criteria used must include information on the implant fixture, the peri-implant soft tissues, the prosthesis and patient satisfaction. Table 2.3b summarises the studies that have reported on success in these different categories, and it is evident that when a comprehensive evaluation of all the criteria that would define success are pooled together, there is a decrease in the reported success rates highlighting the fact that a successful implant has multiple factors that influence the outcome. A surviving implant, on the other hand is one that remains in situ with a history of inflammation, or evidence of infection or complications such as fracture. Survival rates of dental implants range from 89% to 96% over 10 years with 94.6% reported over 13 years with 1.3-mm marginal bone loss. Although the overall implant success and survival rates have been noted to be 88.0% and 97.2%, respectively, bone loss was evident in all 88% of the surviving implants. The reported data on survival and success rates needs to be considered with caution due to the disparate outcome measures used between studies with some reporting success rates of 74% and survival rates of 100%.

A degree of variation is observed between different implant systems and the case complexity with lower survival rates reported in patients with a history of periodontitis and those who smoke. Thus defining success around implants is complex and includes an interchange between implant fixtures (design, surface), patients

Table 2.3a   Criteria for Success as Suggested by Albrektsson et al. 1986.

1.	An individual unattached implant that is immobile when tested clinically
2.	Radiography does not demonstrate evidence of peri-implant radiolucency
3.	Bone loss that is < 0.2 mm annually after the implant's first year of service
4.	No persistent pain, paraesthesia, discomfort or infection
5.	By these criteria success rate of 85% at the end of a five-year-observation period and 80% at the end of a 10-year period are the minimum levels for success

Table 2.3b   Reported Success Criteria for Dental Implant-Retained Prosthesis [1].

Success Criteria	Descriptor	Fixed Complete Prosthesis (six Articles)	Overdenture (five Articles)	Fixed Partial Denture (eight Articles)	Single Crown (10 Articles)
Implant Level	Pain*	4	5	5	7
	Annual bone Loss < 0.2 mm thereafter*	2	3	4	3
	Radiolucency	3	3	5	7
	Mobility*	5	5	6	8
Peri-implant Soft Tissue Level	Probing depth > 3 mm*	2	1	2	2
	Suppuration*	3	3	5	6
	Bleeding	2	0	0	0
	Swelling	1	0	0	0
	Recession	1	0	0	0
Prosthetic Level	Minor complications (chairside approach)	2	0	0	0
	Major complications (failures)	2	0	1	0
	Aesthetics*	1	0	0	0
	Function*	1	2	3	3
Patient Satisfaction	Discomfort/ Paraesthesia*	4	4	1	4
	Satisfaction with appearance*	1	0	4	1
	Ability to chew	1	0	0	0
	Ability to taste	1	0	0	0

* = Most commonly used criteria

(expectations, soft tissue, bone, social and medical history) and operators (experience, knowledge, competence).

Failure of implants is described when the implant, irrespective of the reason, has to be removed or has fallen out. The loss of an implant is multifactorial and includes site-, operator- and patient-related factors. Implant loss of 6% in the first year, 10% in the first 10 years and 12% in the 15 years after surgery has been reported. Table 2.4 summarises the factors affecting implant success rates.

Newer Concepts

As the clinical envelope for tooth replacement has been stretched, the search for newer and more simpler ways of replacing missing teeth in patients with advanced bone loss has been explored. Implant companies are always on the lookout to provide solutions to challenging issues, and the following ideas have been introduced to help overcome some of these challenges especially in patients with advanced bone loss wishing have a fixed solution or a solution that optimises their function and well-being.

- All on 4 or All on 6

This idea was introduced in an effort to help patients with severe atrophy in the posterior regions where there was limited bone or for those who did not want to pursue sinus lift surgery or major bone grafting with onlays. The missing teeth are replaced with a prosthesis that is retained on four or six implants and successful outcomes are dependent on stringent treatment planning. The provision of this type of treatment involves teamwork with the hygienist/therapist being a key member of this team along with the laboratory technician. It is usually considered in patients with all missing teeth, patients with periodontally compromised teeth and extensively carious teeth and teeth that are grossly broken down. The challenge with the concept relates to the patients compliance especially if their teeth have resulted in such a state, how well would they look after their implants.

The philosophy promotes the provision of fixed screw retained prosthesis on the same day for the entire upper or lower jaw following extraction of the teeth and placement of four implants (sometimes six implants) introducing the philosophy of 'teeth in a day'. The dense bone in the anterior part of the mouth is used to place the implants, and the posterior implants are placed at an angle 35–45 degrees to avoid the sinus cavities in the upper jaw and the inferior dental canal in the lower jaw (Figure 2.16). The fixed prosthesis is made from acrylic or composite fused to the titanium, monolithic zirconium or porcelain bonded to a cobalt–chromium frame. Treatment planning is crucial and incorrect planning will result in overload on the implants leading to bone loss and failure. Patient-related factors play a key role and should be considered carefully especially as patients are transitioning from their own teeth to teeth retained on implants. The prosthesis will usually be bulky and speech could be an issue, and parafunction may become a challenge especially in patients who have had teeth that are mobile. As the proprioception around implants is different to that around teeth, patients may generate excessive biting forces without realising it due to the lack of feedback that occurs with teeth that

Table 2.4   Factors Affecting Implant Success Rates.

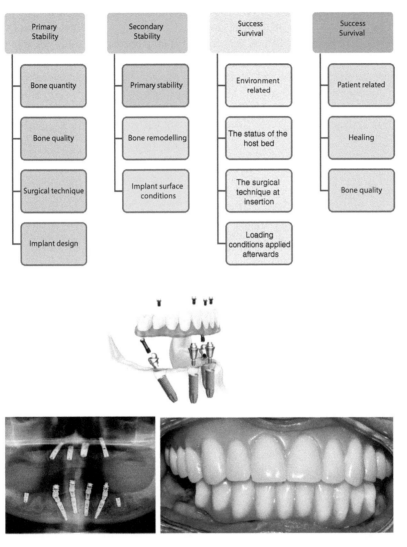

Primary Stability	Secondary Stability	Success Survival	Success Survival
Bone quantity	Primary stability	Environment related	Patient related
Bone quality	Bone remodelling	The status of the host bed	Healing
Surgical technique	Implant surface conditions	The surgical technique at insertion	Bone quality
Implant design		Loading conditions applied afterwards	

Figure 2.16   The all on four concept.

are supported by a periodontal ligament. Thus, these patients will generate higher biting loads resulting in possible fracture and failure especially if the patient has a tendency to parafunction. Whilst successful, with success rates of upto 95% being reported over 10 years, the main complications relate to the unsupported teeth beyond the implants breaking off as a result of excessive stresses and failure of the implants. The philosophy originally introduced by Nobelbiocare, is now offered by all other implant systems within their portfolio.

- Mini Implants

  These implants have been used as an alternative to regular implants where there inadequate bone width. They are a solid one piece screw with a diameter smaller than a traditional implant and can be very thin with diameters of 1.8 mm. The integral ball ended top protrudes out of the gum and can be used to retain dentures and bridges. They are simpler to use and do not have a separate abutment so the restoration is also much easier. As a result the implants are cheaper, however, carry a high failure rate. Due to the size, depending on the use, multiple implants may be needed (Figure 2.17). Their use must be carefully considered against the anticipated outcomes.

Key Learning Points

- Describe the concept of Osseointegration
- Explain the factors that affect Osseointegration
- Discuss the role of different surface
- Interpret challenges they face with implant patients based on underpinning knowledge
- Consider the importance of host-related factors in affecting healing and integration

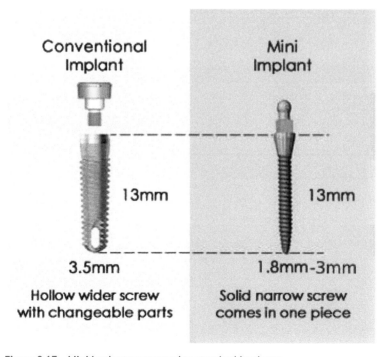

Figure 2.17 Mini implants compared to standard implants.

- Evaluate the parameters of success, survival and failure and be aware of the limitations of published data
- Describe the alternative concepts

References

1 Mohd Axlan Sunil, N., Ashok, and Dharaj. (2015). Criteria for success in dental implants: A systematic review. *International Journal of Scienceand Research* 6: 391.

2 Park, N. and Kerr, M. (2020). Dental implant surfaces. *Dentistry Key*.

3 Albrektssib, T., Zarb, G., Worthing, P., and Eriksson, A.R. (1986). Long term efficacy of currentused dental impalnts – A review and proposed criteriaof success. *The International Journal of Oral & Maxillofacial Implants* 1 (1): 11–25.

4 Albrektsson, T. and Jacobsson, M. (1987). bne-metal interface in osseointegration. *Journal of Prosthetic Dentistry* 57 (5): 597–607.

5 Tagliareni, J.M. and Clarkson, E. (2015). Basci concerpt and techniques of dental impalnts. *Dental Clinics of North America* 59 (2): 255–264.

6 NBarfeie, A., Wilst, J., and Rees, J. (2015). Implant surface characteritis and their effect on osseointtegration. *British Dental Journal* 218: 1.

7 Papaspyridakos, P. and Singh, M. Success criteria in implant Dentistry: A systematic review.

8 Ball, A. and Xia, W. (2011). Dental Implant Surface, physicochemical properties, biological performance and trends Chapter.

9 Park, N. and Kerr, M. (2020). Dental implant surfaces: Dentistry key. Chapter 9, 197.

10 An Do, T., Son Le, H., Shen, Y., Huang, H., and Fuh, L. (2020). Risk factors related to later failure of dental implants – A systematic review of recent studies. *International Journal of Environmental Research and Public Health* 17 (3931): 1.

11 Buser, D., Sennerby, L., and De Bruyn, H. (2000). Modern **implant** dentistry based on osseointegration: 50 years of progress, current trends and open questions. *Journal of Periodontology* 73 (1): 7–21. 2017 Feb.

3

Implant Systems

Implant systems are designed based on the principles described in Chapter 2. Irrespective of the system, the design features aim to provide reduced healing times and rapid integration to provide patients with faster reconstructions. An implant-retained prosthesis is made up of three parts, and each part connects to the other like a piece in a jig saw (Figure 3.1). The precision with which each component is made to fit determines the successful outcome of the restoration. A number of compatible replicas are available; however, it is good practice to use the designated components whenever possible. The growing demand for implants has been driven both by patients and clinicians who are trying to satisfy their patients with manufacturers providing solutions to these demands with newer designs and configurations emerging many of which have little or no published data. A number of the mainstream implant companies have also produced new implant and restorative product lines with limited evidence supporting their success. The focus of these products is to address the demand from patients wanting more rapid solutions for tooth replacement. It is, however, important to remember that these developments cannot overcome the limitations imposed by the biological factors which are integral to successful osseointegration. Whilst every system has specific nuances, making it unique, the majority have features that are common and follow the basic principles related to osseointegration and its success. These features are categorised below.

● Components

All implant systems have four components (described below) that are essential for the provision of implant-retained restorations (Figure 3.2).

A. The Fixture Component (also known as the implant or screw)

This is the part that replicates the root of the tooth and has to be surgically placed into the jaw bone to allow osseointegration into the bone. The different design features and surfaces of the screw that play a role in enhancing osseointegration have been covered in the previous chapter. The screw is designed to facilitate placement into the jaw bone with ease, without causing any trauma to the bone. Some systems have specific designs apically to facilitate atraumatic placement. The top part of the screw on which the prosthesis sits is called the 'platform'. The platform contains the connection into which the prosthesis is connected. The type of connection will influence the marginal bone stability. The

Dental Implants for Hygienists and Therapists, First Edition. Ulpee Darbar.
© 2022 John Wiley & Sons Ltd. Published 2022 by John Wiley & Sons Ltd.

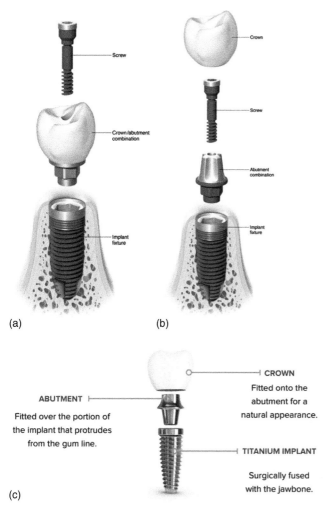

(a) (b)

(c)

Figure 3.1 a, b, c: Component parts of an implant-retained prosthesis (a shows a one-piece screw-retained crown, b shows a two-piece screw-retained crown where the abutment is connected and then the screw connects the crown to the abutment, c shows the abutment being connected and the crown being cemented onto the abutment.

microgap at the platform–prosthetic interface is reported to affect the marginal bone loss; however, if this was shifted medially, then the marginal bone around the implant is noted to remain stable. This concept is called 'platform switching' (Figure 3.3a, b). The junction at which the connection on the platform links the prosthesis to the implant screw, is called the 'implant abutment connection interface'.

This interface is crucial in preventing rotational movement of the prosthesis which usually inserts into the implant screw by the use of either a slip fit or friction fit connection.

There are two main types of connections with different configurations (Figure 3.4). These are:

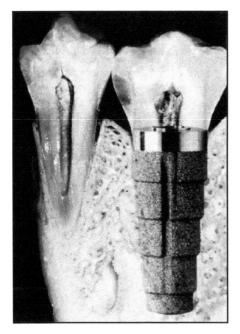

Figure 3.2 Implant screw replicating a tooth root showing the approximation to a natural tooth.

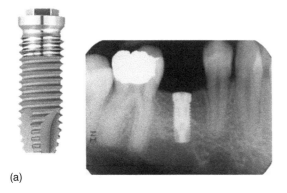

(a)

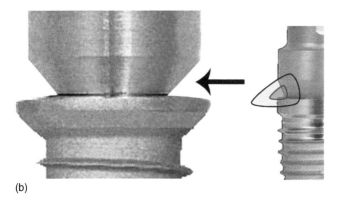

(b)

Figure 3.3 A: Implant fixture (also called a screw). b: Platform switching concept.

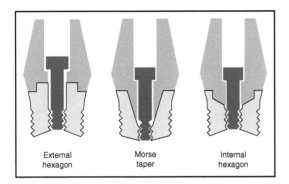

External   Morse   Internal
hexagon   taper   hexagon

Figure 3.4   Cross section of different implant connections.

● External:

This was the first type of connection which protrudes beyond the top of the platform. It is a slip fit connection which can be a hexagon often called the 'external hex' or an octagon with the former being more common. This connection has a higher centre of rotation thus reducing mechanical stability leading to an increased frequency of screw loosening of the prosthesis resulting in its reduced use. Although implants with this type of connection are available, the majority of systems have moved away from this connection due to the stress distribution which occurs largely at the apical area and the marginal area.

● Internal:

This connection sits within the body of the screw. It offers a close and tight fit which prevents micromovement of the abutment, prevents microleakage and distributes forces and mechanical stress generated during function through the body of the implant screw and out towards the bone. There are different internal connection configurations associated with the various implant systems; however, all aim to offer the same function. The configurations include the following:
- the six point hexagon,
- 12 point double hexagon,
- internal cylinder hexagon,
- the trichannel lobe,
- the morse taper design with a mechanically locking friction fit connection with a 5.7° degree or 8° taper and
- the morse taper design with a mechanically locking friction fit connection with a 11.5° cone screw connection.

Figure 3.5 shows the different types of connections.

Although these different connections are used, they do not influence the implant survival or complication rates, however, the internal connection systems have shown slightly lower marginal bone loss. The majority of implant systems today have moved to the internal connection with moderately rough implant surfaces. Table 3.1 shows the connections associated with different implant systems. The surgical technique needs to be modified depending on the connection and is covered in Chapter 5.

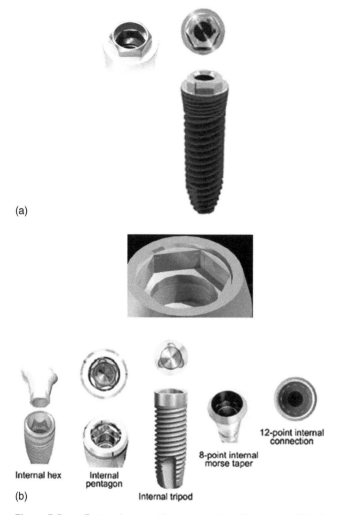

(a)

(b)

Internal hex

Internal
pentagon

Internal tripod

8-point internal
morse taper

12-point internal
connection

Figure 3.5 a: External connection: connection sits on top of the implant platform. b: different internal connection configurations.

B. The Transmucosal Component

This component connects the implant screw into the mouth. It can be a healing abutment which is used to connect the implant screw to the mouth after second-stage surgery or an abutment that will retain and support the prosthesis. The early implants had 'standard abutments' which formed the transmucosal component. The type of implant where the screw part is separate and sits at the level of the alveolar crest and needs a transmucosal component which is either separate or integrated into the prosthesis is called a '2-piece or bone-level implant'. The type of implant where the transmucosal component forms part of the implant screw is called a 'one-piece implant or tissue-level implant' (Figure 3.6). The advantages of the latter relate to the minimal disturbance of the gingival tissues once the implant has been place.

Table 3.1 Connection Types Associated with Different Implant Systems.

Type of Connection	External Connection		Internal Connection	
	Configuration	**System**	**Configuration**	**System**
Slip Fit	External hexagon	Branemark (Nobel biocare)	Internal hexagon	Core Vent
	External octagon	Straumann Narrow Neck	12 point double hexagon	Biomet 3i
	External spline	Calcitek	Internal octagon	Omnilok
			Internal spline	Neoss
			Trichannel lobe	Nobel biocare replace select
Friction fit	Tapered hexagon with 1.5 degree taper	Swede Vent	Internal hex	Zimmer Biohorizon Dentsply Xive
			True Morse Taper (5.7 degree)	Biocon Ankylos
			8 degree cone screw connection (morse taper/ locking taper)	Straumann; Osteo Ti Biomet TG
			11.5 Cone Screw	Astratech
			Conical 5.7 morse taper	Ankylos

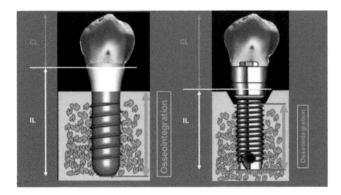

Figure 3.6 Two-piece implant (tissue-level) on the left vs one-piece implant (bone-level) on the right.

- Two Piece (Bone level) Implant types

These systems will usually have the implant screw as one piece and the transmucosal component as the second piece which needs to be connected to the implant screw separately. These implants are placed either at the level of the alveolar crest or slightly deeper. Once the screw is surgically placed, it will either be protected by a cover screw or a healing

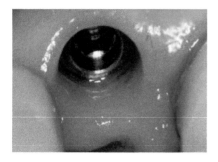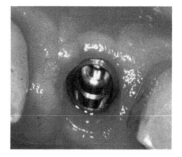

Figure 3.7 Placement of the two (where the implant platform is at the level of the bone) vs one piece (where the implant platform is just below the gingival margin).

abutment. The implant fixture is submerged and covered over by the gum flap and requires a second surgical procedure to expose it and connect it to the mouth through a healing abutment. Increasingly these implants are also being used with the healing abutment being placed at the end of the surgery thus avoiding the need for second-stage surgery. Figure 3.7 shows the healing of the tissues around a 2 piece vs a 1 piece implant with little difference noted in the healing. Once healing has taken place a transmucosal abutment can be used to connect the prosthesis into the implant screw or the transmucosal abutment can be incorporated into the prosthesis and connected as a single unit into the implant screw. The main advantages of the two-piece systems are:

a. Versatility and flexibility especially if there are doubts about the final gingival tissue position
b. Can offer improved aesthetics
c. Flexibility with making custom abutments for the prosthesis

The main disadvantages are:

d. Increased treatment time
e. Need for second-stage surgery
f. Disturbance of the gingival attachment every time the healing abutment is removed

● One-Piece (Tissue Level) Implants

The transmucosal component is incorporated into the implant screw as a one piece. The implant fixture is placed with the top either at the level of the gingival margin or 2 mm below the margin depending on the site in which the screw is being placed. A healing abutment or healing cap is placed to protect the fixture head and thus at the end of the surgery, the metal is visible in the mouth. The key advantages of the one-piece implant are:

g. Eliminates the need for a second surgical procedure
h. Minimises disruption to the gingival tissue seal thereby giving better tissue stability.
i. Simplicity

The key disadvantages are:

j.   Need for careful and considered treatment planning due to the fixed line of angulation with little room to change alignment
k.   Good understanding of the system especially if used in young patients where there is a risk of the transmucosal component to be exposed into the mouth
l.   Potential grey shine through if the gingival tissues are thin

Figure 3.8 shows the issues that can arise if a one-piece implant system is not planned and used correctly. These implants will need to be removed to address the aesthetics as nothing can be done to modify them.

The choice between the one-piece and two-piece implants is purely clinical; however, clinicians should be aware of the limitations of both types when planning their cases so as not to encounter the situation as shown with the case in Figure 3.8. It is therefore important that there is a good understanding of the implant type. Contrary to popular belief if planned appropriately, one-piece implants can be used to restore teeth in the aesthetic zone without any aesthetic risks. Hygienists/therapists should understand these differences as it will affect the peri-implant soft tissue configuration which is an important junction for maintaining health.

● Zygomatic implants

These implants are placed into the zygomatic bone and used in patients with atrophic posterior maxilla or a history of failed sinus lift procedures and failed conventional implants. The different loading protocols covered in Chapter 5 can be used to restore these implants which are used in the posterior regions where there is compromised bone quality with 2–4 conventional implants in the anterior maxilla. They are placed through the alveolar crest and either in the lateral border of the maxillary sinus taking care not to perforate the Schneiderian membrane (intrasinus approach) or outside the sinus called the extrasinus approach (Figure 3.9). The placement of these implants is technique sensitive, requiring a high level of skill with the most common complication being that of sinusitis. Survival rates of upto 96% over 12 years have been reported.

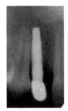
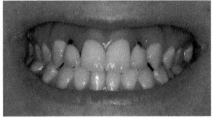
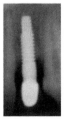

Figure 3.8 A 24-year female has one-piece implants placed when she was 19 years old. The aesthetic compromise is evident where the metal collar is now showing through the gingival tissues which are thin. The radiographs show the incorrect position of the integrated transmucosal abutment in relation to the cementoenamel junction of the adjacent teeth.

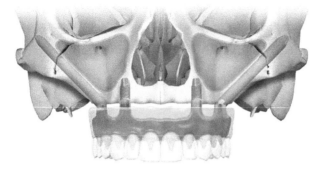

Figure 3.9 Zygomatic implants.

C. The Prosthetic Components

The prosthetic components are very important as they determine the final appearance and the aesthetics which is what the patient will see. The prosthetic components can either be removable or fixed depending on the indication for the implant treatment. They fall into two categories which include the clinical components and the laboratory components needed by the technician to construct the prosthesis. The clinical components include the following:

- Impression coping
  This is a device used to transfer the clinical information about the position of the implant screw and/or the abutment and the soft tissues in the mouth to the laboratory technician. This information can be collected in two ways:
  - At the implant fixture level (called a fixture-level impression)
    Two different impression copings can be used: the pick-up impression coping and the transfer impression coping. In both situations, the impression coping is connected directly to the implant fixture. The main difference is that with the former an open impression tray with holes is used so that the impression coping guide pin juts out of the tray when taking the impression. This is then unscrewed before the impression is taken out of the mouth and the coping comes out in the impression whereas, with the transfer coping, when the impression is removed, the coping stays on the implant fixture and the coping then needs to be unscrewed from the fixture and seated back into the impression taking care to ensure that it has seated completely (Figure 3.10 a, b). The former is called 'the open impression technique' and the latter 'the closed tray technique'. In both cases, it is important to ensure that the coping is connected properly to the implant fixture as any discrepancies will transfer into the final crown. The implant fixture analogue is then connected into the impression copings before the model is poured by the technician giving a replica of what is in the mouth. Transfer impression copings with the closed technique should only be used if there are single units or good alignment of multiple implants. If the implants are divergent, then an open tray technique should be used.

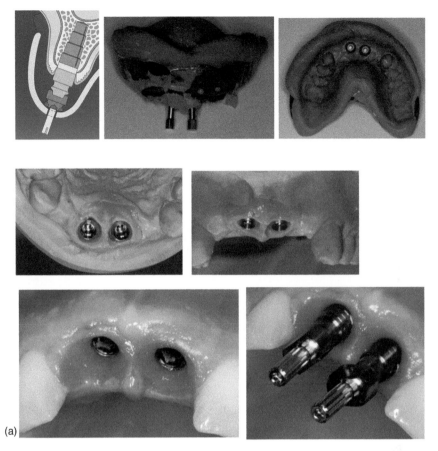

(a)

Figure 3.10   a, b, c: Impression techniques. a: open tray impression with the guide pins protruding from the tray and the working cast poured by the technician providing a replica of what is in the mouth; the pink is the gum tissue replica that the technician creates. b. Impression copings connected in the mouth showing the open-tray technique of a different patient.

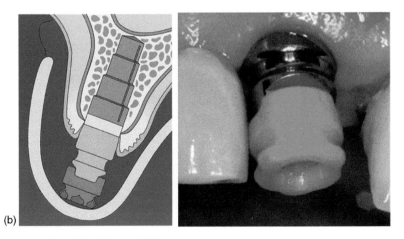

(b)

Figure 3.10b   Closed-tray technique.

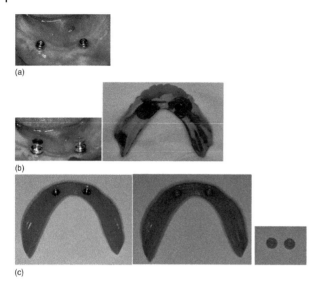

(a)

(b)

(c)

Figure 3.11 a. Abutment level impression with locator abutments in situ. b. With the impression copings in situ and the impression with the copings seated in the impression. b. The technician will connect the fixture analogues to these before pouring the impression. c. Completed denture with the locator caps (pink) inserted into the denture.

- At the abutment level

  The abutment to be used for the final prosthesis is connected onto the implant fixture and torqued to the required level. An abutment level impression coping is connected onto the abutment and the impression taken. The abutment will remain connected to the implant fixture after the impression is removed and protected with a protective cap. The technician will connect an abutment replica into the impression coping before pouring the cast to construct the restoration (Figure 3.11).

● Abutments

An abutment is the equivalent of the body of the tooth onto which a crown or bridge would fit. The type of abutment used will be dependent on the type of prosthesis. Whilst a wide range of abutments are available, for the purposes of simplicity, only an overview of the components will be given so that the hygienist/therapist is familiar with the terminology and can handle any queries from a patient in the midst of their prosthetic treatment presents to them.

The abutment retains the prosthesis on the implant screw and connects directly into it. It can be made as one piece where the abutment is integrated into the prosthesis as one and screwed into the implant fixture with an abutment screw. Alternatively it can be screwed individually into the implant fixture, and the prosthesis is then connected onto the abutment using a prosthetic screw. Abutments fall into three main groups:

- Temporary Abutments

These are used to make a temporary prosthesis.

- Custom-Made Abutments

Custom-made abutments can be prepared to the desired shape by the laboratory technician and have the advantage of delivering the desired shape of the crown. These can also be milled using computer-aided design and computer-aided manufactured (CAD/CAM) technology.

- Prefabricated Abutments

These can be made of titanium, gold or ceramic. They tend to be simple to use requiring little chair-side time; however, the position of the implant screw has to be within the restorative envelop as minimal divergence can be achieved. The choice of the abutment is driven by the type of prosthesis.
Figure 3.12 shows different types of abutments.

- Screws

Screws are used to connect the abutment and the prosthesis to the implant fixture. They are available in titanium or gold, and when used to connect the prosthesis to the implant fixture, is called 'an abutment screw', and the prosthesis to the abutment is called 'a prosthetic screw'. The screws need to be torqued once the prosthesis is connected to minimise the risk of loosening. The abutment screw will usually be torqued to 25–35 NCm depending on the implant system and the prosthetic screw to 10–15 NCm. The prosthetic screws are smaller than the abutment screws which are longer.

- Torque Wrench

These are devices used to apply the required torque to the screws, and whilst previously machine torque drivers were available, today the majority are handheld devices (Figure 3.13). Since the early days of osseointegration, the torque wrench has been made smaller, more versatile and easy to use.

D. Laboratory Components

Laboratory components are replicas of the components in the mouth that the technician uses to construct the prosthesis. They include the following:

a. Implant Fixture Analogue

This is a replica of the implant fixture that is in the mouth. They match all the implant fixture sizes, and the technician will connect this to the impression coping before pouring it to obtain a master model replicating what is in the mouth. The planned implant retained prosthesis is constructed on this.

b. Abutment Replica

This is a copy of the abutment on which the technician will construct the prosthesis. These will be for the preformed abutments.

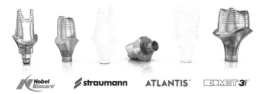

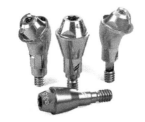

(a): showing the CADCAM range of abutments

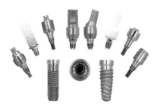

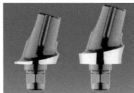

(b): Selection of preformed abutments

(c): Showing the range of Custom and preformed abutments on parallel or tapered implants

Figure 3.12   a, b, c: Range of abutments (CAD CAM milled abutments of the main implant systems and preformed abutments).

c. Retaining Prosthetic Screws

These screws are used in the laboratory during the construction of the prosthesis and are not used to fit the prosthesis in the patients mouth.

d. Gold Cylinders

These are used to make custom abutments so that the crown can be made to match the exact contours required. The prosthesis will be constructed following waxup on these cylinders which have a precise fit into the implant fixtures. Nobel metal alloys are normally used in implant restorations; however, with the price of gold increasing, alternatives with milled metals have been explored.

e. Implant Systems

Currently there are around five mainstream implant systems with published data; however, many of their newer components do not have the five-year data on outcome and performance. Each system has its own unique features which have been modified at different levels covered in the previous chapter to meet the demands from patients and clinicians. Unfortunately, this evolving situation brings different hurdles as many patients who have had the older systems presenting with failures may not necessarily be able to

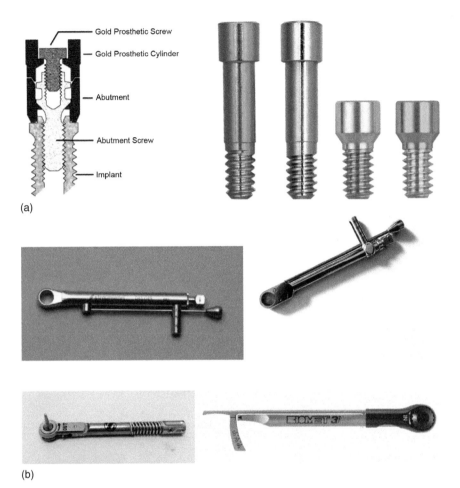

Figure 3.13   a: Gold and titanium abutment and prosthetic screws. b: Different types of torque wrenches.

have these repaired. All systems also offer a wide range of surgical and prosthetic solutions with options available for computer-aided planning and manufacture, implant screw placement and also restoration. These systems are:

● Nobel Biocare (Danahar):

Suppliers of the Branemark implants, although these are largely now superseded by anodised surfaces with design features of the implants enabling shorter healing times and improved stability with internal connections. They also offer the original Branemark-designed implants with external hex connections as well as internal connection more commonly known as 'Replace select'.

● Straumann:

Originally started with their tissue-level implants used as one piece but introduced the bone-level implants to compete with the two-piece implant systems at the same time making use of the platform-switching concept. Their latest implants are made of Ti-Zr alloy with sandblasted and acid etched as well as chemically active surfaces being available. The more recent introduction is the tapered implant within both the bone and tissue-level range with a tapered shape and more aggressive thread pitch.

- Zimmer Biomet

They offer a range of implants which include parallel-sided external and internal hex implants and tapered implants. They are available as either a hybrid implant surface where the top of the fixture is machined or the full surface where the roughness extends to the top of the implant. The implant surface is the osseotite acid-etched surface. Since being bought over by Zimmer, they now have a wider range of implants offering different solutions.

- Dentsply Sirona (Astratech, Ankylos, Xive)

They offer a range of systems which include the previously called Astratech, Ankylos and Xive implants. Each of the implant systems embrace different design features on the implant itself including the type of connection. The implant surface of the Ankylos and Xive implants is an acid-etched surface (cell plus) and that of Astratech is a blasted surface. They also have implants with fluoride on the surface.

- Biohorizons

They offer a range of implants and products but market the 'laser lock' surface which is unique to this system. It provides a positive interlocking attachment between the trans-mucosal abutments and the gingival tissues. The implants are available as one-piece and two-piece implants.

Key Learning Points

- Be able to describe the components of implant systems
- Be able to explain the role of the different components
- Be able to discuss the difference between one-piece and two-piece implants
- Be able to apply knowledge about implant systems to patients who they may treat with different systems
- Be confident in managing patients who may present with problems

References

1 The accuracy of computer assisted implant surgery performed using fully guided templates versus pilot drill guided templates.
2 De Santis, D., Malchiodi, L., Cucchi, A., Cybulski, A., Verlato, G., Gelpi, F., and Nocini, P. (2019). Computer technology applications in surgical implant dentist: A systematic review. *The International Journal of Oral & Maxillofacial Implants* 2014 (29): 25–42. Biomed research international Tahmaseb A, Wismeijer D, Coucke W, Derksen W.

4

Patient Selection and Indications for Treatment

The successful outcome of dental implant treatment is dependent on careful patient selection and risk assessment. This involves a detailed assessment of the patient complaints, their treatment needs and expectations and whether treatment with dental implants will address these. This assessment is even more crucial as the clinical envelop for tooth replacement with dental implants has grown extensively with the focus being on replacing the teeth with implants immediately or within six weeks of extracting the teeth to minimise the extent of bone resorption. Careful case selection and planning is thus the crux of achieving the published success rates with a clear understanding of the limitations of the implant treatment for any specific patient balanced against their expectations. Missing and failing teeth both have a negative impact on the patients quality of life and social well-being; however, this impact is even greater when implants fail with greater consequences on the patients psychological well-being.

The main reasons for tooth replacement are to improve function, aesthetics and psychological well-being as well as maintaining biological structures (e.g. bone and soft tissues) (Figure 4.1). Other lesser reasons may be to help establish other functions, for example, facilitate instrument playing where the front teeth are critical to support the instrument.

Conventional forms of treatment with dentures and bridges provide successful outcomes; however, these are not teeth 'like their own' especially dentures. Thus, whilst any missing tooth can theoretically be replaced with a dental implant, its appropriateness will be dependent on key factors, listed below, that are usually identified during the case assessment.

- Number of missing teeth or teeth to be lost
- The quantity and quality of the soft tissue and bone where the teeth are missing or going to be lost
- The reasons for the tooth loss
- The prognosis of the remaining teeth
- The condition of the rest of the mouth
- The impact of the proposed replacement option on the remaining dentition and oral health

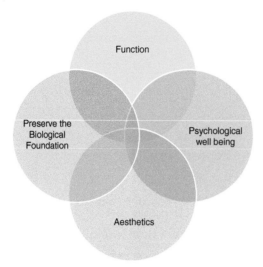

Figure 4.1 Tooth replacement controls the balance of function, aesthetics, psychological well-being and preserving the underlying tissues.

Patient Selection

The process of taking the patient through the journey of tooth replacement enables the clinician to select the patient and their appropriateness to the proposed treatment option. This journey usually incorporates a structured pathway which starts with an assessment of the patients presenting complaints, clinical evaluation and investigations followed by a treatment plan aimed at executing the agreed treatment focussed on addressing the patients' concerns. This journey is critical when dental implants are the preferred treatment option as it will help establish the patients' expectations alongside their compliance to the proposed treatment. It should also take into consideration the clinicians awareness of the dental implant system to be used.

A. Treatment Planning

During this process, the clinician tailors, to the best extent possible, the application of available treatment options and resources to each patient's individual goals and needs. It also includes information about a patient's reasons for seeking implant treatment, their expectations, the goal of treatment, the options for the intervention and possible risks along with the expected length of treatment and factors that could potentially compromise the predictability, long-term success and future maintenance. It should also include information about the costs of the immediate treatment and the long-term follow up and maintenance care that is essential to maintain the outcome after the treatment has been completed.

Treatment planning for an implant patient is undertaken in two phases: the generic phase aimed at primary disease stabilisation and site-specific phase which focuses on the planning for the provision of the implant treatment and includes an evaluation of the site-specific factors (Table 4.1).

Table 4.1 Principles of Treatment Planning for the Implant Patient.

Generic Principles	Site-Specific Principles
Presenting Complaint and History	Revisit the presenting complaint
Medical and Social History	Soft tissues
Extraoral Examination: Smile Line	Periodontal health
Intraoral Examination	Teeth present/absent
Plaque control and periodontal health	Prosthesis
Dentition and state of the teeth; caries;	Missing teeth
Prosthesis	Saddle areas
Occlusion	Gingival tissues
	Bone volume and height
Investigations (Radiographs)	Investigations: wax ups, guides, scans
Diagnosis and Preliminary Treatment Plan	Initial plan – discussion with patient
Primary Disease Management	Finalise the plan
Patient Compliance and Expectations	Treatment outcome

- *Generic Planning*:
The aim of this phase is to establish stability in the mouth and provide the clinician with an opportunity of getting to know the patient and establishing their compliance to advice and guidance given. It is the precursor to the site-specific planning and involves the following steps:

- History
  This enables the framework around which the treatment will be planned and includes four steps:

  - Presenting complaint:
    Establishes why the patient is seeking treatment and the reasons for the tooth loss.
  - Medical history:
    Identifies key issues that may influence the provision of the implant treatment. There are no absolute medical contraindications to implant treatment; however, there are certain conditions that will influence the provision of implant treatment and also affect the long-term outcome to the implant treatment. These include a history of uncontrolled diabetes and hypertension, immunosuppression, oral mucosal disorders and bisphosphonate treatment. Bisphosphonates irreversibly alter the metabolism of the osteoclasts, so there is little or no bone resorption, even if the blood supply is good resulting in osteonecrosis also known as avascular necrosis of the bone or osteochondritis dissecans (the death of bone resulting in the collapse of the bone's structural architecture). This leads to bone pain, loss of bone function and bone destruction. Thus, whilst not contraindicated, the surgical placement of implants may lead to bone necrosis and can also become a long-term complication with symptoms similar to toothache, exposed bone, swelling and altered sensation with recurrent soft-tissue

Table 4.2   Medical conditions that can affect implant treatment.

Moderate to severe neutropenia	Atypical facial pain
Poorly controlled diabetes	Myofascial pain dysfunction syndrome
Long-term corticosteroids	Smoking
Intravenous bisphosphonates	Parafunction
Psychological instability	Cluster phenomenon
Malignancy/terminal illness	

infection. Intravenous bisphosphonate treatment has a greater risk than oral bisphosphonate treatment. A systematic review by Gelazius (2018) reported that patients treated with intravenous bisphosphonates seemed to have a higher chance of developing implant-related osteonecrosis of the jaw; however, the orally treated patient group appeared to have more successful results and thus implant placement in patients treated orally could be considered safe with precautions. Other antihypertensive drugs such as calcium channel blockers will also affect the gingival tissue overgrowth similar to that seen around teeth in the presence of poor plaque control. Table 4.2 gives an indication of the conditions that can affect implant treatment.

- Social history:
  Highlights the risk factors that affect and influence the outcome to treatment both in the short term and the long term. These include the patients smoking history and status and their compliance. Chranovic et al. (2015) have reported that the insertion of implants in smokers significantly affected the failure rates, the risk of postoperative infections as well as the marginal bone loss. Additionally, maintenance of oral hygiene around implants and the risk of peri-implantitis is adversely affected by smoking. Alongside this, stress levels and habits such as parafunction will be established during this step especially as the latter is strongly linked with peri-implant disease.
- Dental history:
  Establishes the patients' attitude to dental treatment and their compliance to protracted courses of treatment.

Throughout these four steps, the clinician will be able to determine the patients expectations and how this aligns with the anticipated treatment with dental implants. It is an important part of the patient management. These four steps are also crucial after the implant treatment when the patient is in the maintenance phase.

- Clinical Assessment

This is undertaken in two steps: the extraoral and intraoral examination.

- Extraoral Examination
  Provides an overview of the features that may influence the aesthetic outcome. These include the facial asymmetry and deviation as well as the profile. The latter will be influenced by the type of implant-retained prosthesis that is being planned. Patients with a history of denture wearing may have lost a lot of bone and replacing a denture with a fixed prosthesis may have a profound influence on the patients' appearance by affecting

the lip support. The smile line at rest and high smile is also assessed to show the amount to tooth on display and how this will affect the end result (Figure 4.2a, b).

- Intraoral Examination

A sequential approach is needed to ensure that factors that could influence the provision of treatment are captured and include the following:

- Soft tissue assessment including an evaluation of the site where the teeth are missing

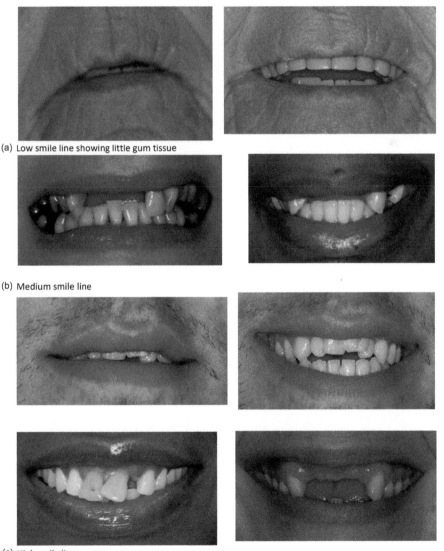

(a) Low smile line showing little gum tissue

(b) Medium smile line

(c) High smile line

Figure 4.2 a: Denture wearer showing the collapse of the lip without the denture (left) and improvement in the support when the denture is worn. b: Different smile lines ranging from low to high.

- Oral hygiene and periodontal health
- Gingival tissues and their health
- Teeth present and the status of the teeth present
- Occlusion including the presence of any teeth that may have drifted
- Prosthesis that is worn

Table 4.3 shows the different components that should be covered under each of these sections.

At the end of this phase, the clinician should have a good understanding of the patients expectations, the challenges they may encounter in delivering the implant treatment both at patient and the clinical level and the possible factors that may influence the outcome to the treatment. Additionally, a rapport will be built with the patient during this phase ensuring that the planned clinical treatment and it possible outcome aligns with what the patient wants. This phase also forms the basis for the long-term maintenance care and follow-up plan that will need to be considered on completion of the active course of implant treatment. During this phase, the need for additional investigations will also be established.

A treatment plan to manage the basic treatment needs including the delivery of oral hygiene instruction and its role as well as stabilizing periodontal disease and dental caries as well as any other interactions should be agreed with the patient and executed before the patient is seen for a reassessment. The hygienist/therapist will play a crucial role during this phase. At this visit, if all primary dental disease has been stabilised, then the patient is ready to embark on the next site-specific planning phase.

- Site-Specific Planning

This phase is undertaken once stabilisation and oral health stability has been achieved. The focus of this phase is to assess the site in which the implant placement is being considered and the adjacent area. It includes an analysis of the following:

- Distribution of the missing teeth or the teeth to be lost, the morphology of the tooth/ teeth being replaced and their relation to the adjacent teeth, the soft tissue and the underlying bone.
- The anatomy and tissue thickness of the edentulous site where the teeth are missing or around the teeth that are planned for extraction.
- Gingival tissue quality: Thin vs thick and the degree of keratinised gingival tissue present.
- Bone quantity and quality which determines the outline form of the ridge and includes the width.
- The occlusion and relationship of the opposing teeth to the site where tooth replacement is being considered.

The assessment will include a combination of visual inspection, palpation and probing. Impressions for study casts and diagnostic wax ups along with additional investigations which may include further analysis of the tissues and radiographic evaluation are also undertaken. These investigations are an important aspect of site planning and allows the patient to become an integral part of the planning and decision making of their treatment which helps ensure that the final treatment plan agreed upon aligns with their expectations making them aware of any limitations mitigating the potential risk of a complaint. Today some of these basic steps can also be performed using digital technology where the site can be scanned and mapped into a file that can be manipulated on the computer.

The gingival tissue quantity and quality, referred to as the biotype, is evaluated visually and using a probe. The biotype is described as thick or thin and is usually challenging to establish as most patients will present with tissues that are a combination of the two types. Thick tissues are usually 'fibrous looking' and thus easier to note (Figure 4.3), Although a number of methods have been advocated to assess gingival tissue thickness, their application is limited due to the significant variation between individuals. The simplest way of assessing gingival tissue thickness is through the use of a probe and the degree of grey shine through when the sulcus is probed (Figure 4.4). The quantity of gingival tissue relates to the extent of attached gingivae, also called keratinised tissue present (Figure 4.5). Its depth varies and can range from 0 mm to 12 mm in height. The absence of keratinised tissue around teeth and implants has been associated with a higher risk of inflammation. With dental implants, this higher risk of inflammation is due to the nature of the mucosal attachment to the transmucosal abutments. Soft tissue augmentation techniques can be used to change both the quality and quantity of the gingival tissues and are covered in chapter 5.

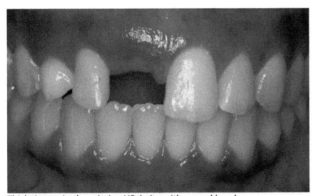

Thick tissues in the missing UR 1 site with a good band of keratinised tissue

Mixed gingival tissue biotype which is predominantly think with recession and minimal keratinised tissue

Figure 4.3   a, b: Gingival tissue biotype – thick vs thin tissue.

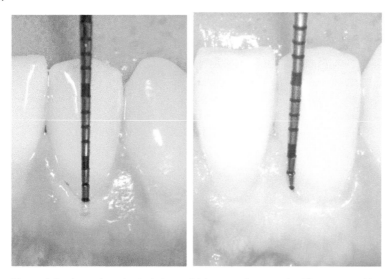

Figure 4.4 Assessing gingival tissue thickness using a probe. The grey markings of the probe shining through the thin gingival tissues is clearly visible. In contrast where the tissue is thicker (right picture) this is not so obvious.

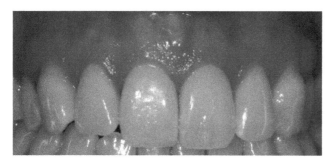

Figure 4.5 Anatomy of the gingival tissues in health showing the stippling with keratinised tissue.

The bone volume (width) and height is assessed first by visual observation and palpation. Different techniques have been employed to measure the quantity of bone and include ridge mapping (also called bone sounding). In this method the proposed implant site is anaesthetised and the depth of the soft tissue measured at intervals. This data is then transferred onto a sectioned stone cast in the same alignment as the measurements were taken and the markings joined giving an outline of the bone width and height (Figure 4.6). The information collected is used with conventional periapical radiographs of the site. Whilst the use of conventional radiography is beneficial during the generic planning, site-specific planning using three dimensional multislice computerised tomograms introduced in 1993 give a detailed preoperative evaluation of the bone quantity, quality and adjacent anatomical structures in relation to the planned prosthesis, the outline of which is translated to the scan through a radiographic guide also known as a stent. Radiographic guides, replicating the anticipated position of final tooth, are usually worn when the teeth are missing prior to

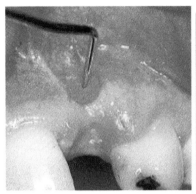
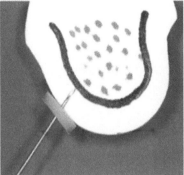

Figure 4.6 Bone/ridge mapping using sectioned casts.

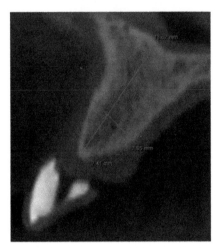

Figure 4.7 Cone beam scans showing the radiographic template in situ mapped against the bone present.

the scan being taken to show the underlying bone in relation to the tooth. This will help establish whether there is enough bone to place the implant in the restoratively driven position and the need for augmentation and when it should be carried out. Implant planning software that matches the data to the diagnostic wax up information enables the clinician to view the planned implant position in relation to the bone quantity and planned prosthesis and establish the need for adjunctive bone grafting and possible risks. More recently cone beam computerised tomograms which reduce the level of radiation exposure have changed the way three dimensional implant planning is undertaken with computer-guided static and dynamic surgical implant placement being used to minimise risk (Figure 4.7).

The minimum bone volume needed for predictable and safe implant placement is reported to be 4–6 mm for a standard implant diameter of 4 mm and bone height of 7–9 mm with a minimum distance of 1–2 mm between the adjacent teeth and dental implants with a variation of 1 mm depending on the type of tooth being replaced and the diameter of implants being used. These dimensions are today, general reference guides, since the evolution of bone

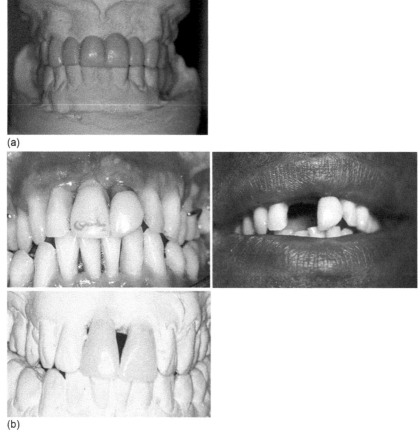

(a)

(b)

Figure 4.8 a, b: Conventional diagnostic wax ups showing the changes in tooth position that can be achieved. a shows multiple teeth that need to be modified and b shows the anticipated change that could be achieved and the possible difficulties that may be encountered. In this case the patient was unhappy of the aesthetics and the wax up was used to show that the UL 1 would have to either be modified or removed and that he would have a space in between the teeth even if the contact point was improved.

augmentation and grafting techniques and the use of short and wide implants. These along with the changing technology and improved understanding around osseointegration has changed the way we plan dental implants pushing the clinical envelop such that the use of shorter and wider implants has almost become routine practice. Irrespective of the bone width and height, an implant fixture should have primary stability at placement to obtain the best outcome and precise preoperative planning remain the crux of successful treatment.

Study casts with diagnostic wax ups (Figure 4.8) are invaluable during the planning of implant treatment allowing an assessment of the site to be examined in different angles as well as offering the following:

- Establishes the shape, size and position of the teeth which will assist in the choice of implant diameter

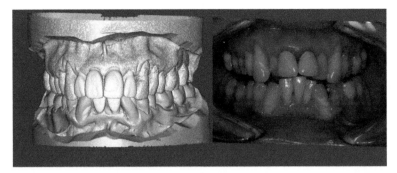

Figure 4.9 Virtual diagnostic wax ups showing the improvements in tooth shape and position. The virtual wax up allows the patient to visualise the planned tooth position.

- Shows the intended end point of the planned treatment when shown and discussed with the patient along with the possible challenges
- Highlights potential issues that may affect the aesthetic result
- Gives a visual assessment of the interocclusal and intraocclusal space available from different angles and the occlusion
- Used to construct the radiographic and surgical guides once the tooth position has been confirmed
- Can be made as a fixed or removable prosthesis. The latter can be worn by the patients giving them a true representation of what the planned prosthesis would look like

The conventional ways of constructing study casts and wax ups have now been superseded by digital technology where the impressions taken of the teeth can be scanned to construct three-dimensional virtual representation of the mouth with virtual wax ups alongside the planned occlusion. These images provide an opportunity of giving the patient a real feeling of what the planned prosthesis would look like (Figure 4.9).

At the end of the site-specific planning, the clinician will be able to explain to the patient the treatment needed for the execution of the implant treatment, the time it will take and the anticipated outcome. This communication ensures that the patient has a good understanding of and is familiar with what is being considered and planned and what can be achieved with the implants. They also have the opportunity of raising issues or concerns they may have before any irreversible treatment is undertaken. It is also important that any shortcomings to what the patient wants and their expectations of treatment are highlighted and discussed at this time.

The final part of the treatment planning will conclude with an indication of the maintenance care regime that the patient will need to follow and the time intervals based on the risk analysis undertaken. The patient being an integral part of the process should understand what is being planned from the outset and their role in ensuring that the long-term successful outcome.

Figure 4.10 shows the process map of the paitents journey from start to finish and Figure 4.11a–f shows a patient going through this journey.

Today, with advances in digital technology, digital impressions can be taken of the teeth and transmitted to the laboratory for the manufacture of virtual models, with the pathway taking the patient through a digital journey right from the start of the planning stages to the execution of the treatment and the construction of the prosthesis and its fit.

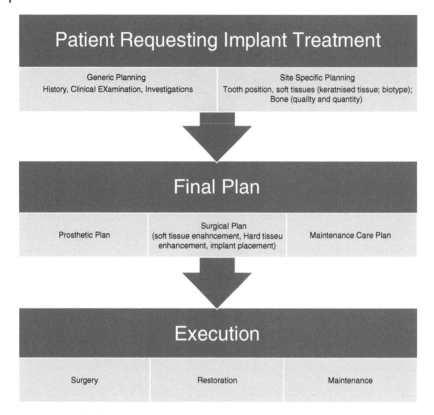

Figure 4.10   Patient journey from presentation to completion of treatment.

Indications for Implant Treatment

Tooth loss is considered as a public healthcare issue and despite the multiple preventive measures, its incidence remains high. Dental implants are one of many tooth replacement options and are not suitable for everyone. Therefore, when considering tooth replacement, the conventional options of tooth replacement with dentures and bridges should not be overlooked. The generic phase of the planning will help establish the reasons for the tooth loss and whether dental implants would be an appropriate option. The main reasons for tooth loss are:

- Periodontal disease
  Severe periodontal disease affects upto 10% of the population worldwide and remains one of the most common causes of tooth loss. Patients who have lost their teeth due to periodontal disease are not poor candidates for dental implant treatment; however, it is essential that existing periodontal disease has been treated and stabilised before any consideration to tooth replacement with dental implants. The prognosis of the remaining teeth should also be considered and contingency planned to future loss if the teeth are to be retained. Patients who have lost their teeth due to periodontal disease will often

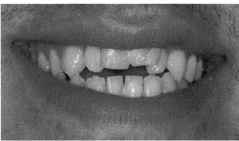

(a): Preoperative view showing low smile line and poor appearance. He wanted to improve his appearance especially the UL 1.

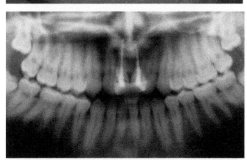

(b): In occlusion showing poor plaque control and inflammation with poor tooth position of the UL 1 and UR 1: Generic plan was to establish gingival tissue health and removal of the UL 1 which had a poor prognosis.

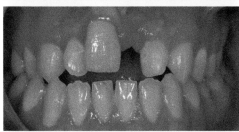

(c): Orthopantomogram showing the UR 1 and UL 1 both root filled with UL 1 having resorption. Prognosis is deemed to be poor.

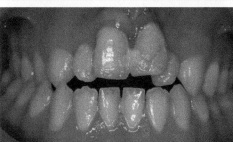

(d): Post initial phase therapy and extraction of UL 1 with limited space; Short term tooth replacement was with a denture. Orthodontic treatment was planned after further hygienist treatment; Site specific planning indicated lack of space and the ideal space was discussed with the orthodontist.

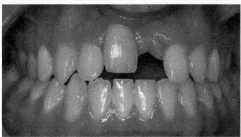

(e): Post orthodontic treatment with good oral hygiene and healthy gingival tissues; UR 1 was ankylosed and could not be moved; Final Planning: A diagnostic wax up was undertaken to establish the tooth position and what could be achieved with the UR 1 in situ. This was discussed with the patient with ongoing maintenance care and the surgical plan driven by the position of the final prosthesis that was agreed upon.

Figure 4.11 a–h: Show a patient following the journey outlined for the replacement of his incisor tooth with a dental implant.

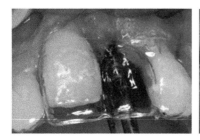
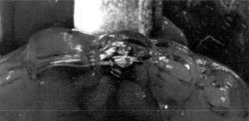

(f): Surgical placement of the Implant Fixture with surgical guide in situ showing the fixture position to replicate the ideal tooth position; UR 1 was left in situ due to the low smile line and ankylosis and age of the patient who was in his 20's; The fixture was placed using a tissue level fixture as one stage.

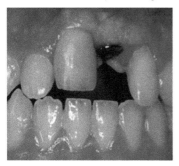
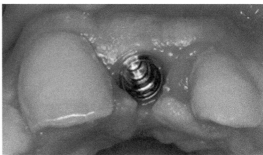

(g): Fixture insitu at the time of impression taking. UR 1 has been prepared to receive a veneer to improve the aesthetics (agreed during the final planning); Note marginal plaque on the mesial of the UL 2 and the need for ongoing maintenance care.

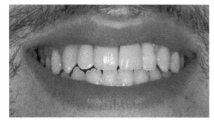
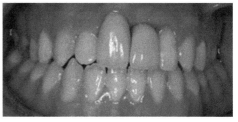

(h): Final prosthesis which was a veneer on UR 1 and cement retained implant crown on UL 1 showing the excellent aesthetics; The higher gingival margin of the UR 1 was not an issue as the patient had a low smile line. The patient is now on a 3 monthly maintenance care plan.

Figure 4.11 Continued

present with soft and hard tissue loss with complex treatment needs and careful treatment planning is essential to ensure success. Patients who have had the periodontal disease treated and are well motivated have been shown to have successful implant treatment outcomes, although when compared to non-periodontally susceptible patients, the success rates are slightly lower with upto 85% reported over eight years. These patients will need stringent and regular follow up and maintenance care on completion of the implant treatment as they remain at a higher risk of peri-implant disease.

- Dental caries
  This is the second-most-common cause of tooth loss. The overall caries risk needs to be evaluated as this will influence the prognosis of the remaining teeth. The need to contingency plan future loss of teeth that have a compromised prognosis in relation to the implant treatment is essential to ensure a positive outcome.

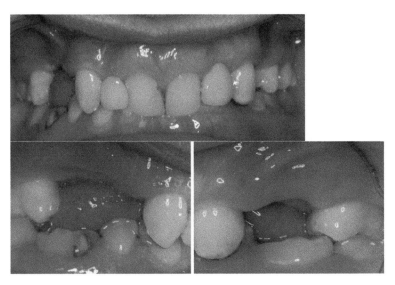

Figure 4.12   Patient with hypodontia showing the issues with bone volume and tissue type.

- Endodontic failure
  Success rates of endodontically treated teeth remains high; however, often teeth that are endodontically treated will fail either due to recurrent infections apically or due to root fracture. If replacement of these teeth with dental implants is planned, it is crucial to ensure that the infected tissue is entirely removed to ensure the outcome to implant treatment remains favourable. Implants placed in sites with a previous history of recurring apical infections may be at a higher risk of failure, and those placed adjacent to endodontically compromised teeth are also at risk and thus planning should factor the prognosis of the adjacent teeth in these situations.

- Dentofacial trauma
  Traumatic injuries to the teeth affect ~ 20% of the population during their lifetime. The injuries can be varied and localised to the teeth alone or involve the soft tissues, bone and facial structures. The challenges associated with replacing the missing teeth is dependent on the injury and those with extensive tooth tissue loss will need a multidisciplinary approach to care. When the injury is localised to the teeth only, replacement of the teeth with dental implants will offer a more favourable option providing psychological benefits and improved quality of life.

- Congenital absence
  The prevalence of patients born with missing teeth remains relatively high and can occur independently or as part of a syndrome. Patients with congenitally missing teeth will often have other anomalies with lack of adequate space, quality of the gingival tissue and quantity and quality of bone (Figure 4.12), thereby needing additional integrated interventions to create the required shape, form and space for the teeth to be replaced with dental implants. In these patients, the treatment expectations are usually underpinned by emotion which often needs to become part of the treatment planning process.

Table 4.3 Components that should be considered during the Intraoral Examination

Component	Parameters to be Assessed	How
Soft tissues	Mucosa Salivary flow	Visual
Ridge defect	Quality Size Width and heigth Concavities	Visual Probes Other investigations
Periodontal health	Oral hygiene Gingival tissues –Biotype – Keratinised tissue Bleeding Probing depths	Visual Probe
Teeth present	Number Restorations Caries Tooth wear Overeruption Drifting	Visual Probing Other investigations
Occlusion	Discrepancy in retruded / intercuspal position	Visual
Prosthesis	Fixed vs removal satisfactory	Visual, probing handling

- Implants used to facilitate other treatment

  Dental implants are increasingly being used to provide anchor for orthodontic tooth movement when natural teeth are compromised. The implants can either be in the form of mini tads or conventional implants. If the latter are used then the position of placement should be planned such that the implants are in the required position at the end of the orthodontic treatment and can then be restored.

- Follow-Up Care

The maintenance regime and anticipated follow-up care the patient will need should be considered during the generic and site-specific planning phases. The maintenance care regime will be dictated by the risk indicators and predictors and will also be influenced by the type of prosthesis. Planning of the prosthesis should be such that it facilitates the patients plaque control thus maintaining tissue stability and health.

The follow-up intervals will be dictated by the patients compliance and manual dexterity as well as their understanding on how to look after their implants. The follow-up protocol and timings should be considered and thought about during the planning so that the patient is fully aware that implant treatment requires a commitment for life.

A balance against the indications for the tooth replacement against the stringent measures used to select the patients will help inform the type of prosthetic reconstruction and the surgical techniques used to facilitate the implant treatment. At the end of treatment planning phase, the clinician and the patient both should have an understanding of the anticipated end point, the surgical and prosthetic steps needed to achieve this end point alongside the mitigating factors that could influence it with the expected follow-up periods. Furthermore the patient at the end of this stage will have a better appreciation of their role in achieving a successful outcome not just during the treatment but also on completion of the treatment.

Key Learning Points

- Explain the importance of establishing patient expectations
- Discuss the steps involved in treatment planning
- Describe how the preoperative planning defines the maintenance care regime
- Consider the indications for treatment and how they impact on decision making
- Appreciate the importance of the generic phase in planning for implant treatment
- Explain the role of site-specific implant planning and the value of the soft tissue and bone quality and quantity and how it influences outcomes
- Explain the patient journey during implant planning and understand how decision made during this journey could influence provision of maintenance care

References

1 Bryington, M., De Kok, I.J., Thalji, G., and Lf, C. (2014 Jan). **Patient** selection and **treatment planning** for **implant** restorations. *Dental Clinics of North America* 58 (1): 193–206.
2 Zitzmann, N.U., Margolin, M.D., Filippi, A., Weiger, R., and Krastl, G. (2008). Patient assessment and diagnosis in implant treatment. *Australian Dental Journal* 53 (1): S49–59.

5

Surgical and Prosthodontic Protocols

Surgical and prosthodontic treatment protocols are underpinned by well-performed pre-operative examination and planning which helps ensure that the expected end result is achieved. It is the fundamental basis upon which the surgical and prosthodontic protocols are built and treatment executed. Whilst we describe the 2 separately, both aspects of dental implant treatment are integrated and have to be considered together during the planning phases with the surgical plan being driven by the expected prosthetic solution known as 'crown down planning'. The diagnostic wax up will enable the construction of surgical guides that should be used during the surgical implant placement to ensure that the orientation and position enable the provision of the restoration as per the original treatment plan.

Surgical Protocols:

These are shaped by a prosthetically driven plan which shows the type, shape and morphology of the planned tooth/teeth position usually aided by a diagnostic wax up covered in the previous chapter. The protocol includes the surgical assessment plan and the surgical intervention.

- Surgical Assessment

Aspects of the surgical assessment will have been covered during the generic and site-specific planning phase. The patients' compliance, attitude to surgical treatment, their suitability and ability to cope with surgical treatment should have been established during this phase along with the following:

  - medical conditions that may affect the surgical intervention and post-surgical healing e.g. uncontrolled diabetes, haematologic disorders (such as haemophilia) which increase risk of bleeding during and after surgery
  - smoking history which, if the patient is a smoker, may affect the surgical intervention and flap handling as well as the outcome to the surgery due to the compromised vascularity
  - patients' ability to tolerate lengthy procedures
  - mouth opening to facilitate instrumentation especially towards the back of the mouth

- proximity of local anatomical factors e.g. nasopalatine canal, sinus floor, inferior dental canal, root proximity of the adjacent teeth in the vicinity of where the implant fixture is to be placed

If one or more of the above parameters are deemed unsuitable then caution should be exercised in proceeding with surgery as it will compromise the outcome to implant treatment and place the patient at risk. If the factors are deemed suitable then surgical intervention is planned and undertaken.

- Surgical Intervention

The aim of surgical intervention is to provide access to the site and facilitate all the procedures needed to ensure the prosthetically driven placement of the implant fixture facilitating the provision of the final restoration. The site being planned for surgery should be healthy with no signs of inflammation. The principles for surgical intervention include:

- atraumatic site access which will include the flap design determined by the type of implant placement and the need for augmentation.
- atraumatic site preparation with no overheating of the bone, the use of sharp drills at slow controlled speeds using copious irrigation and no pressure to avoid overheating the bone aiming for primary stability of the implant fixture.
- maintaining a safe distance of at least 2 mm between the implant fixture and anatomical structures.
- placing the implant fixture within the restorative envelop as defined by the surgical stent.

Timing of Implant Fixture Placement

The standard placement of an implant fixture submerged for six months has now become extinct due to the advances in the understanding of post-extraction bone resorptive changes, implant fixture design and surface topography. The timelines in which implant fixtures can be placed are:

- Immediate placement at the time of extraction (called Type 1 placement):
  This requires a higher level of understanding and planning to minimise the complications that could occur as a result of the post-extraction bone resorptive changes. If the bone quantity is inadequate to allow the correct positioning of the implant fixture with primary stability, then immediate placement should not be considered.
- Early implant placement at four to six weeks after extraction (called Type 2 placement):
  Allows soft tissue healing prior to implant fixture placement.
- Delayed placement at 12–16 weeks after extraction (called Type 3 placement):
  Allows soft tissue healing and some bone healing to be complete prior to the implant placement. However, if the bone volume is inadequate for primary stability then a staged approach where the bone volume is re-established with augmentation first should be considered.
- Late or conventional placement at four to six months or more (called Type 4 placement):
  The site is allowed to heal for a period of four to six months following extraction prior to implant placement. It is usually considered if there is lack of primary stability of the implant fixture using the previously described techniques. Standard implant placement is applied to edentulous sites.

Table 5.1 shows the different timings for fixture placement. These options allow improved predictability by reducing the degree of bone loss and by creating stability of the soft tissues. Type 2, 3 placement are the most common type of approach used today. The timing of implant placement is further defined by the loading protocols using A, B, C to describe the type of loading that has taken place. This is covered later in this chapter.

● Flap Design

Different flap designs have been used to place dental implants and the choice is determined by the need for augmentation at the time of implant fixture placement. Flapless designs whereby a flap is not raised but access obtained either via the extraction socket when the tooth is removed, or through the use of a soft tissue punch have been advocated but are technique sensitive and should be carefully planned (Figure 5.1a,b,c). The flapless approach is generally used with a computer-guided surgical approach covered later. Other designs include the use of 2-sided or 3-sided flaps with relieving incisions to improve access. These flap designs enable coronal advancement if augmentation is anticipated. Pouch incisions which give exposure to the site are also used but are more common when augmentation is not needed or around extraction sockets. Irrespective of the flap design, the basic principles in relation to flap handling and maintaining the blood supply as well as ensuring that the required access is obtained should be observed. Poor access to the surgical site will lead to complications and potential implant failure. In sites where augmentation is needed, the flap design should be such that it enables periosteal release for coronal advancement of the flap. The flap at all times when replaced should be passive and not under tension.

Table 5.1 Timelines for Dental Implant Placement.

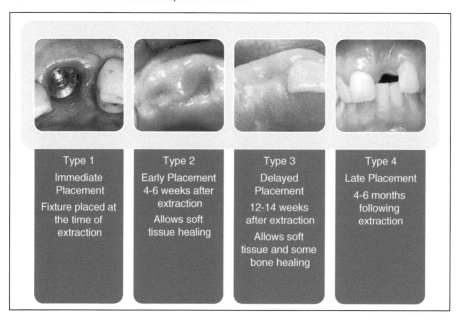

Type 1	Type 2	Type 3	Type 4
Immediate Placement	Early Placement 4-6 weeks after extraction	Delayed Placement	Late Placement 4-6 months following extraction
Fixture placed at the time of extraction	Allows soft tissue healing	12-14 weeks after extraction Allows soft tissue and some bone healing	

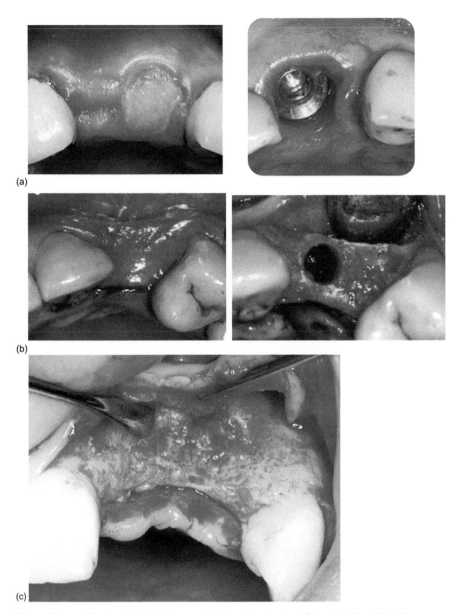

Figure 5.1 a: Flapless implant placement where the implant fixture is placed into the extraction socket without raising a flap. b: Crestal incision with a pouch-designed flap raised to place the implant screw. Note the palatal position of the incision to maintain the keratinised gingival tissue. c: One-sided flap raised for implant placement and simultaneous augmentation.

- Site Preparation and Implant Fixture Placement

Once the bone has been exposed, it is essential to ensure that the procedure is completed within the shortest time possible to minimise unnecessary bone exposure. The site should be managed carefully and all granulation tissue removed. The site is prepared using an incremental drilling sequence with the final drill being slightly smaller than the implant fixture itself. This enables the primary stability of the fixture to be achieved. Figure 5.2 shows the drilling sequence leading to implant fixture placement. In sites when the bone is very dense i.e Type 1 bone, tapping the site with a screw tap would be needed to facilitate the placement of the implant fixture to reduce the risk of overheating the bone. In contrast, sites where the bone is very soft i.e. Type 4 bone, will need a modified approach with the final osteotomy being prepared using bone condensers to expand the site to the required dimensions or stopping 1 drill short of the final drill before the implant fixture is placed. The techniques used aim to ensure osteotomy preparation with minimal trauma such that stability of the fixture can be achieved. Once prepared, the implant fixture is installed using either machine driven or handheld instrumentation. The placement torque can range from 20 NCm to 50 NCm; however, torques higher than 50NCm should not be used due to the risk of damaging the bone. The installed fixture is protected either with a cover screw or a healing cap/abutment before the gum flap is replaced and sutured in place, the choice of which will be dependent on the degree of augmentation needed. Figure 5.3 a–f shows the site preparation and final implant fixture placement.

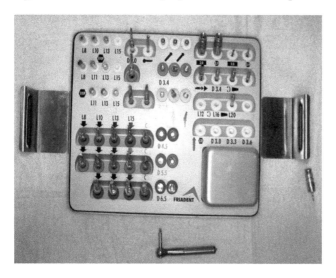

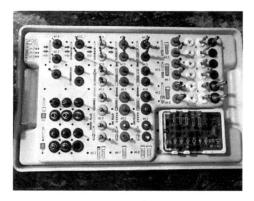

Figure 5.2 Surgical tray showing the drilling sequence for implant fixture placement.

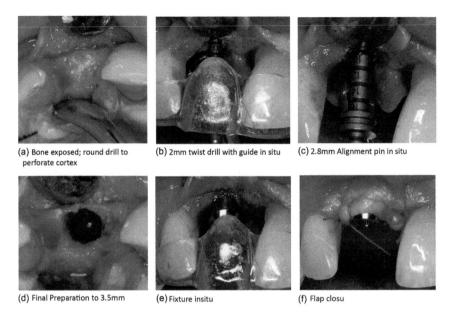

(a) Bone exposed; round drill to perforate cortex

(b) 2mm twist drill with guide in situ

(c) 2.8mm Alignment pin in situ

(d) Final Preparation to 3.5mm

(e) Fixture insitu

(f) Flap closu

Figure 5.3   a–f: Drilling sequence for the one-piece implant placement (protocol will vary with different systems, but they all follow the same steps – perforate the cortex, incremental stepwise widening of the osteotomy site and final drill smaller than the implant diameter. The sequence is showing placement of a 4.1-mm fixture diameter.

- Type of Implant Fixture Placement

As covered in Chapter 2, implant fixtures, depending on the type of the system, and whether they are one or two piece, can be placed using a two-stage or a one-stage approach. In the former, the implant fixture after placement is submerged under the gum flap and protected using either a cover screw or a healing abutment and in the latter a healing abutment is used immediately after the implant fixture placement allowing the gingival tissues to mature around the healing abutment. With the two-stage approach a minor second surgical procedure is needed to connect the fixture to the mouth (Figure 5.4). The decision regarding the type of fixture placement will be made during the planning phase and will be determined by the degree of primary stability and the extent and type of augmentation needed at the time of placement.

Computer-Guided Placement

Computer-guided static and dynamic virtual implant surgery has been used with the former being more commonly used. In this type of surgery, virtual planning of the optimal implant position aligned with the future prosthesis is undertaken using interactive planning software which superimposes this position onto the cone beam computerised scan. This information is then translated into a tissue- or a tooth-supported drill guide with mechanical positioning devices fixed to the jawbone to facilitate the preparation of the osteotomy and the implant fixture inserted in the predicted ideal position thus providing the best possible outcome in relation to the prosthetic design, aesthetics and occlusion. In contrast dynamic virtual surgery also known as navigation, uses visual imaging tools on the computer monitor and

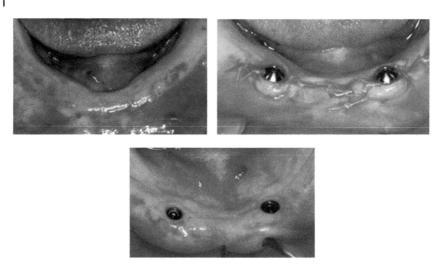

Figure 5.4 Second-stage surgery to expose the implants (before, after exposure, after healing).

specialised equipment to navigate the surgery and the implant fixture position both of which can be altered if needed in real time. It allows both virtual surgical guidance and virtual implant fixture placement. Both techniques require a degree of skill and experience.

Augmentation Procedures

Augmentation is defined as a procedure that is undertaken to enlarge or maintain a body part. When applied to dental implantology, it refers to the procedures undertaken to enhance or maintain the soft (gingival) and hard (bone) tissue quality and quantity. The need for augmentation and its timing will be recognised during the site-specific planning phase and the timing and type of augmentation needed finalised during the surgical assessment if optimum outcome to the implant treatment is to be achieved. Augmentation procedures should not be left to chance and need careful planning for predictability. Major augmentation is undertaken when the bone and tissue loss is severe and extensive grafting is needed to re-establish both. Such procedures will usually involve grafts that are taken from the iliac crest (hip bone) and need to be undertaken by a trained maxillofacial surgeon. Major grafting is not undertaken in the dental surgery and is not covered here although the patient may be seen in the dental practice setting for their maintenance care.

Augmentation undertaken in the dental surgery, is called minor augmentation, and can be undertaken prior to the placement of the implant fixture, at the time of the implant fixture placement or after the implant fixture placement during the early healing period or at the second stage surgery phase or during the maintenance phase (Figure 5.5). Its need will be determined by the gingival tissue biotype and the presence or absence of keratinised tissue and the width and height of bone present to facilitate the prosthetically driven implant fixture placement and includes either soft tissue augmentation only, bone augmentation only or a combination. Fifty to sixty per cent of the population present with either fenestrations and/or dehiscences around the teeth thus indicating that the majority of patients who lose teeth will have some form of bone deficiency necessitating augmentation (Figure 5.6).

At the time of extraction (socket preservation)
Before implant placement (staged)

- Socket anatomy
- Soft tissue quantity and quality
- May involve both soft and hard tissue

At the time of implant placement (simultaneous)

- Must achieve primary stability of the implant
- Defect anatomy
- May involve both soft and hard tissue

After the placement of implants

Figure 5.5 Different timings for augmentation to facilitate implant fixture placement.

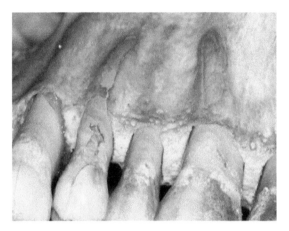

Figure 5.6 Skull showing the fenestrations and dehesicences on the buccal aspect of teeth.

Timing of Augmentation

● Soft Tissue Augmentation

The aim is to either increase the amount of keratinised gingival tissue or increase the thickness of the gingival tissue. The importance of the gingival tissue quality and quantity around implants influences the long-term stability and as a result the treatment outcome. The influence of these tissues is due to the anatomical variation of the mucosal attachment around the transmucosal abutments covered in Chapter 6.

Keratinised tissue has been shown to reduce the risk of peri-implant inflammation by providing stability and forming a tight cuff around the gingival margin and the transmucosal connection. The lack of keratinised tissue results in tissue movement resulting in plaque accumulation and inflammation (Figure 5.7). The gingival tissue biotype has been shown to influence aesthetics and thick tissues are more resistant to trauma and thus offer improved stability around dental implants. It also determines the risk during the maintenance care of peri-implant disease and the patients' ability to optimise the cleaning in the area.

The soft tissue profile is determined by the underlying bone. Soft tissue augmentation can be undertaken:

- Prior to the implant fixture placement
  This will be done to enhance the keratinised tissue or the tissue thickness or both and aims to enhance the soft tissues prior to the implant placement. The removal of muscle attachments which may affect the flap stability during the implant fixture placement can also be undertaken at this time (Figure 5.8a).
- At second stage surgery after the implant fixture placement
  If the soft tissue looks compromised and is thin, soft tissue augmentation can be undertaken to increase the tissue volume thickness. Keratinised tissue augmentation may also be needed at this time (Figure 5.8b).
- After the implant placement during the maintenance phase
  In sites with lack of keratinised tissue or tissue thickness where there is inflammation indicative of peri-implant mucositis/peri-implantitis (Figure 5.8c).

O Hard Tissue (Bone) Augmentation
  As the aesthetic demand for tooth replacement has grown, the placement of implants where the bone is present without any consideration of the final tooth position has long gone. This along with the need for maintaining biological health and functionality has resulted in augmentation techniques being used to facilitate

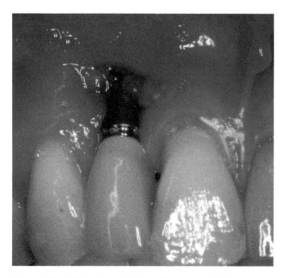

Figure 5.7 Thin gingival tissue biotype with tissue movement due to lack of keratinised tissue causing plaque accumulation and inflammation.

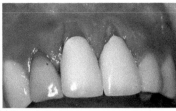
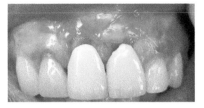

(a) Before implant placement a connective tissue graft has been used to increase both the tissue thickness and keratinised gingival tissue.

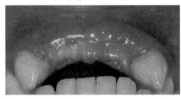
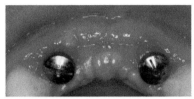

(b) At second stage surgery a porcine matrix has been used to increase tissue volume

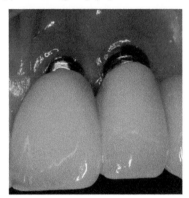
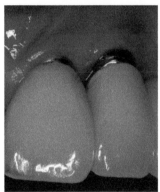

(c) After implant placement, a connective tissue graft with an epithelial collar has been used to increase thickness and keratinised tissue

Figure 5.8 a–c: cases showing soft tissue augmentation undertaken at different timelines.

the prosthetically driven placement of implant fixtures. Hard tissue augmentation follows the principles of guided bone regeneration where the epithelial and connective tissue cells are excluded to allow the bone cells to grow (Figure 5.9). It can be undertaken at the following times:

○ Prior to implant fixture placement in healed sites where teeth have been previously extracted and the remodelling process has resulted in compromised bone volume and height which needs to be re-established to facilitate the implant fixture placement. This is called the 'staged' approach and a healing period of four to eight months is usually needed before the implant fixture placement depending on the materials used for the augmentation (Figure 5.10a).

○ Prior to implant fixture placement in extraction sockets
Following tooth extraction, bone loss occurs both horizontally and vertically, with the majority of changes seen within the first eight weeks. The horizontal bone loss ranges from 29% to 62% and the vertical loss ranges from 11% to 22% with the degree of bone loss being influenced by the presence of infection, trauma and anatomy as well as the

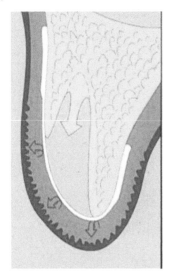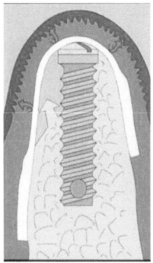

Figure 5.9 Principles of guided bone regeneration: Barrier is used to selectively exclude unwanted cells from infiltrating into the defect allowing the required cells, in this case bone to grow. Table 5.2 shows the types of barriers used for guided bone regeneration.

technique of extraction. Thus, when teeth are extracted, these resorptive changes reflect the residual shape of the edentulous ridge. Augmentation at the time of extraction is recommended to minimise the extent of bone loss seen following extraction. Although it does not stop the post-extraction bone remodelling changes, it helps reduce the amount of augmentation needed subsequently at the time of implant fixture placement. This is also called 'socket preservation'. Preserving the socket will not stop the bone remodelling and loss but will minimise the extent of the bone loss seen (Figure 5.10b).

○ At the time of implant fixture placement known as 'simultaneous' augmentation. The implant fixture placement will be determined by the surgical stent thus ensuring that the position of the fixture is in the prosthetically determined three-dimensional alignment. Augmentation at this time will facilitate the aesthetic end result. When the augmentation is undertaken to improve the horizontal bone volume, it is called 'contour augmentation' (Figure 5.10c).

○ After the implant fixture placement
This is usually during the maintenance phase when augmentation may be undertaken to regenerate bone lost as a result of peri-implant disease. This will not recreate osseointegration as the implant surface will already be a contaminated implant surface (Figure 5.10d).

Techniques for Augmentation

Techniques such as distraction osteogenesis whereby fracture of the bone is surgically induced and the two parts pulled apart slowly allowing bone growth over time and revascularised grafts, where the vital bone segment is transferred to its recipient bed with its vascular pedicle, most commonly used in cancer surgery are used to increase bone height

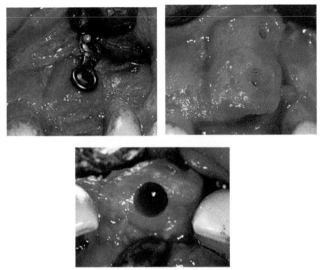

(a) Staged approach where a block graft of autogenous bone is used to increase the bone volume facilitating implant fixture placement. The picture on the left shows the graft in situ with the fixation screws, after being removed and the graft prepared to receive an implant fixture.

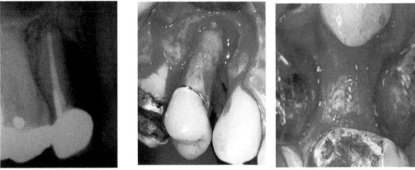

(b) Hopeless tooth extracted and socket preserved showing the bone volume was maintained at 4 months re-entry into the site.

Figure 5.10 a–d: Cases showing hard tissue augmentation undertaken at different timelines.

and width. However with both these techniques general anaesthesia is needed and thus is not undertaken in the dental chair.

The technique of guided bone regeneration is the most commonly used technique and involves the use of a barrier for selective cell exclusion allowing bone formation into the space created (Figure 5.9). Bone defects for augmentation are described as space making and non-space making and often graft materials are used to preserve or help create the space in conjunction with barriers, which selectively exclude the unwanted cells, allowing the bone cells, to grow into the defect. These techniques are used to reconstruct deficient ridges both vertically and horizontally using a combination of block or particulate grafts depending on the defect anatomy. The main goal for augmentation to work predictably is to have wound stability during the healing phase as any micromovement will lead to fibrous tissue formation. When undertaken simultaneously during implant placement, primary stability of the implant fixture is needed.

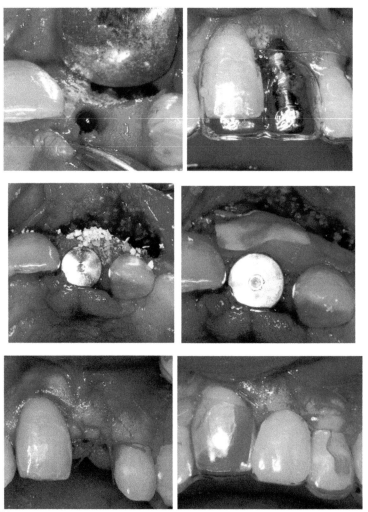

(c) Simultaneous augmentation (same case as seen in Chapter 4) at the time of implant placement using a 1 sided flap approach. An Essix retainer is used to ensure that there is no trauma to the underlying site.

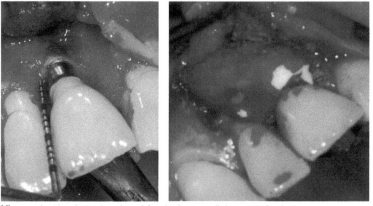

(d) Peri-implantitis with mesial intrabony defect that has surgically been treated with augmentation

Figure 5.10 Continued

Other techniques such as ridge splitting/expansion using specialised instruments are undertaken to increase the volume (width) in sites where the ridge is thin and bone width is compromised. Horizontal augmentation to increase the width of the ridge is also called contour augmentation and is more predictable than vertical augmentation where height of bone is needed. Vertical bone height can be gained by undertaking sinus lift procedures in the maxilla or onlay grafts. In the former, it is important to identify the position of the final restoration in relation to the adjacent teeth prior to this being done as usually an onlay graft would give a more aesthetic result.

Materials for Augmentation

- Soft Tissue

The materials used for soft tissue augmentation can be grouped into autografts, allografts, and xenografts (Figure 5.11). The autografts (connective tissue and free gingival) remain the gold standard providing optimal predictability; however, challenges with second site surgery and quantity available has led to the use of alternative materials. Whilst the outcome to treatment of the materials used is similar, the allografts and xenografts show a greater degree of contraction shrinkage during the initial healing periods; however, avoid the need for second site morbidity and being off the shelf products quantity is not an issue. Figure 5.12 a–d show the use of the different materials.

- Hard Tissue/Bone Augmentation

Augmentation of the bone heals by the following principles:

- Osteoinduction: whereby new bone cells are induced through the use of growth factors or bone morphogenic proteins
- Osteoconduction: whereby the grafting material serves as a scaffold
- Osteoproduction: whereby the grafting material dissolves encouraging the formation of bone
  There are different materials used for bone augmentation and can be categorised into the following groups (Table 5.2):

- Autogenous:
  This bone is obtained from the same individual. These grafts have the highest predictability and can be used as blocks or particulates. They can be taken from extraoral donor sites (major augmentation) and intraoral sites such as the chin, ramus or tuberosity. They remain the gold standard as they have a combination of both osteoinductive and osteoconductive properties; however, challenges with rapid resorption has led to the use of these grafts in combination with the other materials to slow down the resorptive process.

- Allografts:
  These are obtained from another individual of the same species also called cadaveric bone. The material is available as freeze-dried bone allograft and decalcified freeze-dried bone allograft and live tissue. They have largely osteoconductive properties and outcomes are variable depending on the bone bank from which the material was obtained.

Table 5.2 Barriers Most Commonly Used for Guided Bone Regeneration; All Ideally Need to Be Used with a Grafting Material.

Type of Barrier	Category	Comments
Non-Bioabsorbale	Titanium shield (Frios)	Need to be stabilised
	Titanium Mesh	Can be CAD-CAM manufactured
	Polytetrafluoroethylene Based (ePTFE- Goretex;	ePTFE can get exposed and infected
	dPTFE – Cytoplast)	dPTFE is more tissue friendly
	PTFE – TefGen-PD	
	Titanium reinforced available to offer stiffness	
Bioabsorbable	**Collagen Based**	
	Bovine (Type 1 collagen)	
	Biomend; Collaplug	Varying degrees of stiffness but all need to be used with a graft material
	Porcine	
	Memlok Pliable (Type I)	Can be fixed
	Creos (Porcine and Elastin	Exposure triggers early absorption
	Biogide (Type I + III collagen))	Handling properties vary between the different types
	Pericardium	Bioabsorption rate varies from four to six months and some show longer periods
	Memlok (human pericardium)	
	Synthetic (polylactic -PLA and polyglycolic- PLG acid based)	Bioabsorption times variable
	PLA: Guidor	Need stabilisation
	PLA/PLG-Cytoflex resorb	

- Xenografts:
  These are animal-based materials obtained from either cows (bovine), pigs (porcine) or horses (equine). Algae- and coral-derived materials are also available based on calcium carbonate formulations. All the materials are processed stringently through structured processes aimed at reducing disease transmission. The quality of the grafting material will vary depending on the porosity with porcine bone having the highest porosity. The materials are available in different particle sizes with the small ones used for the small defects. The materials are osteoconductive and provide the scaffolds for the bone formation.

- Alloplasts:
  These are synthetic materials which are grouped as hydroxyapatite, calcium phosphate derived, calcium sulphate derived and bioactive glasses. These materials are also osteoconductive and used as defect fillers with variable-handling properties and resorption rates. The bioactive glasses, in contrast, have been reported to be osteoproductive as they have been shown to stimulate bone formation. Hydroxyapatite has been shown to heal by fibrous encapsulation. The use of synthetic materials is variable and whilst successful have a limited evidence base.

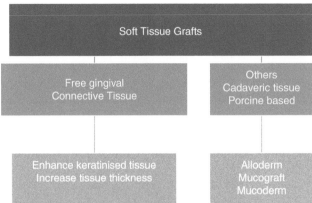

Figure 5.11 Different types of soft tissue grafts.

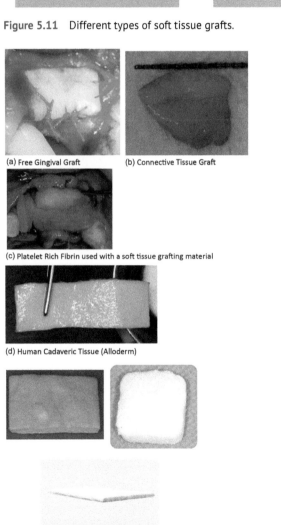

(a) Free Gingival Graft   (b) Connective Tissue Graft

(c) Platelet Rich Fibrin used with a soft tissue grafting material

(d) Human Cadaveric Tissue (Alloderm)

(e) Porcine Based Materials (Mucograft, Fibrogide, Mucoderm)

Figure 5.12 Different materials used for soft tissue grafting.

  − Growth factors:

  These are osteoinductive and include plate-rich plasma/fibrin and bone morphogenic proteins. The former is used increasingly in implant dentistry with successful outcomes and is often mixed with the materials mentioned above.

Autogenous bone remains the gold standard due to its superior properties with osteoinduction and conduction. However due to challenges with second site morbidity and quantity, autografts are often used in conjunction with one of the other materials. The xenograft materials are the most popular due to the ease of availability and predictability. Synthetic materials also have a place in the market for people who do not wish to have animal products (Figure 5.13 a–c).

  The outcome of the augmentation is related to the type of defect and site being treated as well as operator experience. Grafts are often used in conjunction with barriers to prevent the downgrowth of the epithelial cells which can lead to fibrous union as opposed to

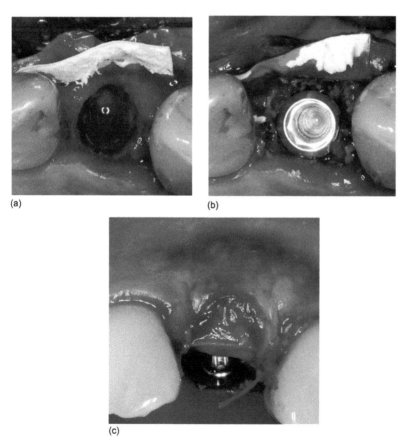

(a)

(b)

(c)

Figure 5.13 a–c: Immediate implant fixture placement with simultaneous augmentation. The barrier is placed on the buccal aspect where there is a fenestration. The site is prepared and implant fixture placed and the gap augmented using a biomaterial. The healing cap is placed and the flap closed over.

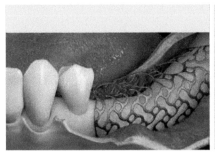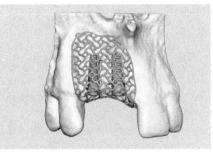

Figure 5.14 Computerised titanium framework used as for space maintenance.

integration. Table 5.3 gives an overview of the types of barriers with the resorbable collagen barriers being the most popular due to their ease of use. However, these barriers lack stiffness and thus need to be used in conjunction with a hard tissue grafting material to maintain the space for the bone regeneration. With advances in computerised technology, customised titanium frames can be made to maintain space and used with the collagen barriers to facilitate both horizontal and vertical regeneration (Figure 5.14).

Table 5.3 Different Graft Materials Used for Augmentation.

Type of Graft	Description	Comments
Autogenous (Humans)	Block Graft	Second site needed
	Particulate	Quantity
		Resorption rates
		Often used with other materials
Allograft (Other Humans)	Freeze-Dried Bone Allograft (FDBA)	Outcomes variable
		Remain in situ for long times
	Decalcified Freeze-Dried Bone Allograft (DFDBA)	
Xenografts (Animal Based)	Bovine	Most commonly used
		Different types depending on the provider and thus have variable outcomes
	Porcine	More porous
	Equine	
Alloplasts (Synthetic)	Hydroxyapatite	Defect fillers and often heal with granulation tissue
	Bioactive Glass	Can stimulate bone production but variable
	Calcium Phosphate and Carbonate Based	High resorption rate
Others	Platelet-rich plasma (PRP) and platelet-rich Fibrin (PRF)	Variable outcomes reported
	Bone morphogenic proteins	Expensive

Prosthodontic Protocols

The prosthesis is what the patient will see at the end of the treatment and thus it needs to be designed to meet the patients' functional and aesthetic needs. Thus giving the patient an indication of what this could look like at the outset is really important to ensure patient engagement with the process but also to manage their expectations. It will also enable the clinician to ensure that the expectations align with what is realistically feasible within the clinical envelope, e.g. patients wanting a fixed prosthesis when they have been long-term wearers of a removable prosthesis will need to be aware of the aesthetic compromise due to the compromised lip support related to the bone and tissue loss. The prosthodontic protocols aim to define the type of implant-retained prosthesis that is to be provided to the patient as well as ensuring the occlusal scheme that will be adopted. The latter is crucial and plays a significant role in minimising the early and late complications often seen after the fit of the prosthesis. Some of the early complications with the technical aspects of implant prosthetic failures e.g. screw loosening have been overcome by the changes in design and technology. The design and type of prosthesis will determine the long-term prognosis and success of the implants as it will match the patients' ability to maintain the implants e.g. a patient with poor manual dexterity may struggle to clean around a fixed prosthesis and thus either the design may need to be changed or a removable prosthesis considered.

The planning of implant treatment should always begin with the end in sight and should be the first consideration given when looking at tooth replacement with dental implants. The generic planning phase will help with understanding the patients' wishes and expectations, and these views can be taken into consideration during the site-specific planning. This early planning will aid the clinician into understanding the number and size of the implants and their distribution which will depend on the number of teeth missing and the degree of bone and soft tissue loss.

The choice between a removable prosthesis and fixed prosthesis should be made at the beginning especially if a patient wearing dentures is seeking a fixed alternative to achieve these treatment goals. The majority of patients want teeth that are fixed in their mouth; however, the provision of such a prosthesis will be dictated by a number of factors covered later in this chapter. The goal of the prosthetic treatment will be determined by the patients' needs and functional status. At this time the clinician will also need to engage with an experienced and well-informed technician who will be responsible for the construction of the prosthesis. The clinician should be able to communicate with the technician and translate the anticipated vision so that the final prosthesis meets the requirements and expectations of the end point. This communication has become simpler with the introduction of digital technology with the conventional methods of constructing a prosthesis being supplemented by the computer-aided design- computer aided manufacture (CAD-CAM). This has made some of the more challenging laboratory aspects of providing implant-retained restorations simpler.

Prosthodontic protocols therefore focus on ensuring that the patients' expectations are balanced against predictability of what can be achieved within the clinical constraints. They should include the following:

- Type of prosthesis: fixed or removable
- Design of the prosthesis should maintain health i.e. facilitate cleaning

- The material of which the prosthesis is to be made
- Type of retrievability
- Occlusal scheme

Type of Prosthesis

Implant-retained prosthesis are either removable or fixed. A hybrid prosthesis is one which utilises the soft tissues for support and the implants for retention. The choice between the two options will be dependent on the degree of soft and hard tissue lost as well as the patients' manual dexterity which is an important factor to consider for maintenance. The removable prosthesis will replace both soft and hard tissues and can be of a hybrid design or solely retained by the implants. Fixed prosthesis can replace a single tooth (crown) or multiple teeth (bridges) or all the teeth. When all the teeth are to be replaced with a fixed implant-retained prosthesis, retrievability and a contingency plan for future failure should be considered especially if the prosthesis is to be made as a single unit. A fixed prosthesis will be able to replace some soft tissue and requires a greater degree of manual dexterity and aftercare and may be associated with higher maintenance costs.

- Removable Prosthesis

  This type of prosthesis aims to enhance retention, stability, and function and is removed by the patient for cleaning. It is used when there is extensive soft tissue loss that cannot be replaced with a fixed prosthesis and will have a detrimental effect on the facial profile and ultimately appearance. There are four different attachment systems used to retain the denture on the implants. These are:

  - the ball/stud/locator attachments,
  - bar attachments,
  - magnets and
  - telescopic attachments.

Locator abutments have superseded the use of the ball/stud attachments. The choice of attachment is dependent on the interocclusal space, patient-related factors and clinician choice. Figures 5.15a–c show the different types of attachments used.

The construction of the denture will follow the same principles as constructing a conventional denture. Dentures retained on implants are called overdentures and usually two implants are advocated in the mandible and four in the maxilla when such a prosthesis is planned. Patients must be made aware of the need for minor adjustment after fit and also the need for regular maintenance and follow up. A common complication around bar-retained dentures is reactionary hyperplasia that is often seen under the bar. Remake of implant-retained dentures is usually needed around ten years or sooner if the patient has a tendency to parafunction; however, depending on the wear and occlusion, the retaining inserts of the attachments may need to be replaced within a couple of years.

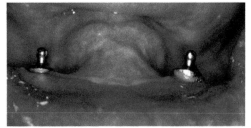

(a) Ball ended abutments: These are largely superseded by locators

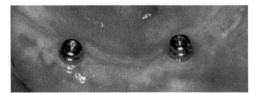

(b) Locator abutments used to retain denture

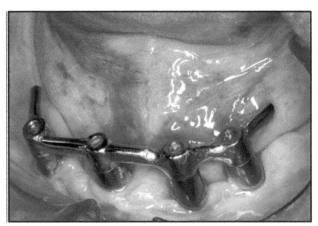

(c) Bar attachments; Manual dexterity is needed for cleaning under
the bar. It gives more rigid fixation to the denture

Figure 5.15 a–c: Ball ended, bar and locator attachments for implant overdentures.

- Fixed Prosthesis

This type of prosthesis is fixed to the implant either directly using an abutment screw, or indirectly via an abutment in which the latter is first connected to the implant with the abutment screw and the prosthesis is either connected via the abutment with a prosthetic screw or cemented onto the abutment (Figure 5.16). This type of prosthesis cannot be removed by the patient. The abutment screws are usually preloaded by being torqued at the time of fit to 25–35 NCm and prosthetic screws to 15 NCm depending on the implant system being used. The access hole through which the screw is connected has to be sealed off and before the filling material is placed, the head of the screw is protected using tape or cotton wool before the filling material is placed (Figure 5.17). Screw-retained restorations tend to be more bulky than cement-retained restorations. Advances in technology and digital systems have made it possible to have angle correction screws which allow minor angulation changes to be made in the prosthesis. These screws need special drivers. Cemented

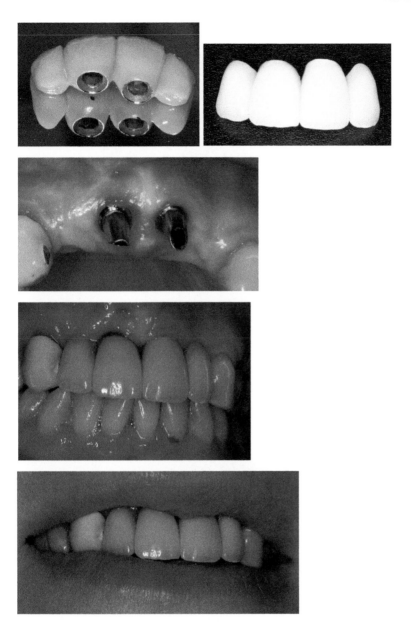

Figure 5.16 Fixed cement-retained implant prosthesis.

implant restorations usually use temporary luting agents to allow retrievability. Temp bond with modifier has been a popular cement; however, challenges with removing the excess cement and retrievability has led manufacturers to develop special cements for cementing implant-retained restorations (Figure 5.18). These cements based on resin formulations, have a 'snap set' which allows removal of the cement minimising the risk of cement-induced peri-implant inflammation. Due to the precision fit of the prosthesis only a small amount of cement is needed. Cement-retained restorations and crowns overall offer better

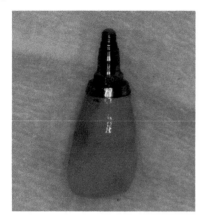
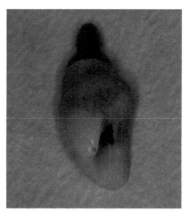
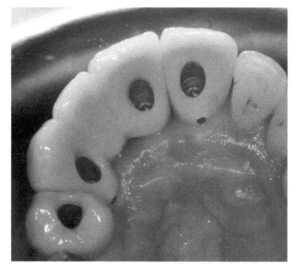

Figure 5.17 Access hole of a screw-retained prosthesis.

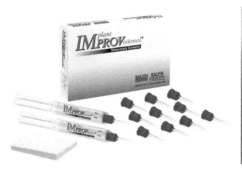
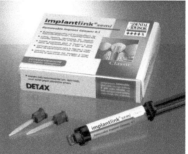

Figure 5.18 Resin-based cements used for cementing implant restorations.

contours aligned with the natural teeth. There is no unanimous consensus agreement about the type of restoration; however, screw-retained prosthesis should be considered when multiple units, full-arch frameworks and situations where retrievability is crucial.

Complications Associated with Implant-Retained Restorations

Prosthetic complications usually are technical complications and are related to occlusal forces and the design of the prosthesis. These can be grouped into minor and major complications as follows:

- Minor:

Screw loosening, fracture of the prosthetic material, decementation, loss of the screw access hole filling and wear (Figure 5.19a–c)

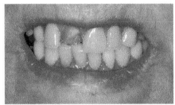
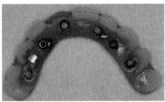

(a) Tooth debonded off the prosthesis due to wear and tear leading to occlusal instabilty

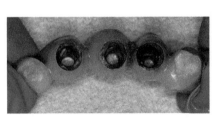
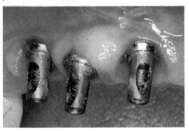

(b) Decementation of a cement retained bridge that had been in place for more than 5 years. The abutments are preformed abutments

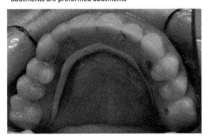

(c) Loss of the screw access hole filling; this needs to be replaced to stop food debris getting caught into the holes.

Figure 5.19 a–c: Minor complications associated with implant-retained restorations.

- Major:

Screw fracture, framework fracture and implant fracture (Figure 5.20a, b)

Depending on the nature of the complication, a simple repair can be undertaken; however, the clinician must assess the reasons for the complication and rectify this otherwise the progressive deterioration can lead to a minor complication becoming a major one.

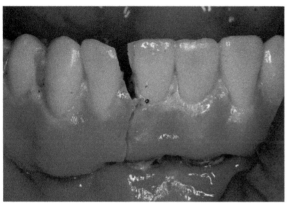

(a) Fractured Prosthesis

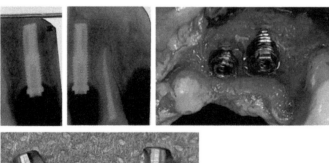

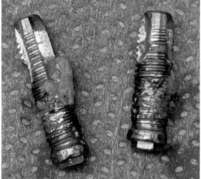

(b) Fractured abutment screw inside the implant which led to the implant having to be explanted as the screw could not be removed. The implants had been in situ >10 years.

Figure 5.20 a, b: Major complications associated with implant-retained restorations.

Loading Protocols for Implant-Retained Restorations

The control of the occlusion and the occlusal scheme used is an important part of ensuring that adverse loading forces are controlled and the stresses distributed favourably to minimise the risk of technical or biological complications. The loading protocols around implants have evolved over the last few decades and contrary to the early days of implantology, where the implant, once placed was not loaded for four to six months, are now being loaded earlier and earlier. Some of these changes are driven by the improved designs and surface topography of implants. The loading protocols currently used are:

● Immediate loading:

The prosthesis is connected to the implant fixture within one week of implant placement and is in occlusion with the opposing teeth. This protocol should only be applied when there is excellent primary stability and augmentation has not been undertaken.

● Early loading (sometimes referred to as delayed loading)

The prosthesis is connected to the implant fixture within one week to two months of implant placement

● Conventional loading

This approach is used when the implant is left to integrate into the jawbone for at least two months or more with no connection to the prosthesis and the prosthesis connected after this period of integration.

● Immediate Restoration

The prosthesis is connected to the implant fixture but is kept out of occlusion with the opposing teeth and is usually fitted within one week of implant placement.

The choice of these loading protocols will be dictated by the degree of primary stability, the need for augmentation and the soft tissue stability. In cases where the implant is left to heal for a period of time, the temporary prosthesis has to be tooth supported to minimise trauma to the underlying tissues and implants. Inadvertent trauma from the temporary prosthesis can lead to early implant failure.

Constructing the Prosthesis

The prosthesis can be delivered at time of implant placement (called immediate restoration), after four to eight weeks of implant placement (called early restoration) or after three months (called conventional restoration). Immediate restoration is usually undertaken when aesthetics is of concern and stability of the implant has been obtained but is not ready to be loaded. Irrespective of the type of prosthesis the construction of the implant-retained prosthesis follows the same steps described below. The number of steps needed will be dependent on the number of implants and the type of prosthesis.

● Impressions

These are taken either at the time of the implant placement or after a healing period depending on when the restoration is to be fitted. These can be taken either at the implant fixture level or at the abutment level. For the latter the abutment has to be connected to the implant fixture first and the appropriate impression coping used to take the impression. Fixture-level impressions are taken using an open tray when the screw retaining the coping protrudes out of the tray or closed tray when the screw is covered within the impression and a transfer cap is connected on the top (Figure 5.21). In the former, the coping has to be unscrewed before the impression is removed and when taken out, the coping remains in the impression. In contrast, with the closed technique, the clinician has to remove the impression coping and replace it into the impression. Some systems have a pick-up version of the closed tray. The details of the different impression copings and abutment types have been covered in Chapter 2. The impression is disinfected and sent to the laboratory for the next stages. All implant systems will have components that follow similar steps.

Digital technology has enabled conventional impressions to be scanned onto digital software from which the laboratory constructs the prosthesis. Digital impressions can also be taken using digital scanners and remove the inconvenience of messy impression materials, are easier for patients to tolerate and minimise the need for sending stuff to the laboratory as the images taken are transmitted to the laboratory digitally using specialised software. Digital impressions require the use of a coded healing abutment or a scan body which provides reference markers that the technician will use on the digital image to construct the prosthesis (Figure 5.22).

● Laboratory Stages:

Depending on the type of impressions taken, after disinfection, the technician will connect the fixture analogue to the impression coping and the impression will either be poured or scanned. If there is a wax up and a guide, this will be used to construct the final prosthesis;

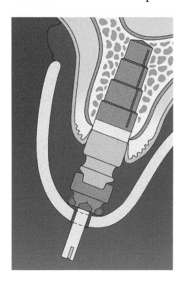 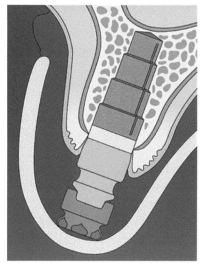

Figure 5.21   Impression techniques – open and closed tray (covered in Chapter 3).

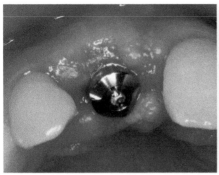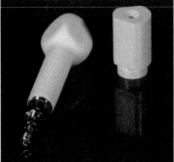

Figure 5.22 Encode abutment and a scan body used for digital impressions.

however, for digital scans, the images of the wax up are mapped onto the impression for the prosthesis to be constructed. For multiple implants with bridges where a framework is needed, this would be tried in the mouth first and verified before the final prosthesis is manufactured. A bisque bake try-in of the prosthesis is undertaken when there are shade match challenges or the contour of the prosthesis needs to be established.

Fitting the Prosthesis

Once the completed prosthesis is received from the laboratory, the clinician will check the fit on the cast and assess the prosthesis. The healing abutments are removed and the prosthesis tried into the mouth. For multiple custom abutments, a transfer jig is used to ensure the correct alignment of the abutments to facilitate seating of the prosthesis (Figure 5.23). The abutments are connected and the screws torqued. The prosthesis is fitted to the framework with either cement or screw. For the former, prior to cementation, the access holes are sealed off to prevent the cement getting caught into the access holes. The framework must have a passive fit on the implants to ensure no traumatic forces are transmitted to the underlying implants. The occlusion is checked and the patient given advice on the aftercare and function. Patients may be referred to the hygienist/therapist for this guidance.

Radiographs and post-fit periodontal charting are taken at the time of fit of the prosthesis as they will form the baseline reference from which to assess the periodontal tissues and the bone levels during the first few years.

Post-Insertion Instructions

Depending on the type of prosthesis, the instructions given to patients are crucial as they will need to look after their prosthesis. Before the patient leaves they should be:

- Shown how to clean around and under the prosthesis if it is a bridge
- Informed about the importance of daily and optimal cleaning
- Shown how to use different tools for the cleaning

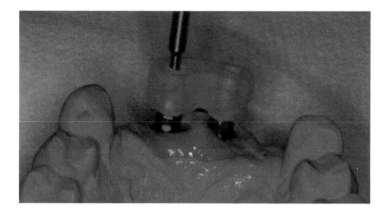

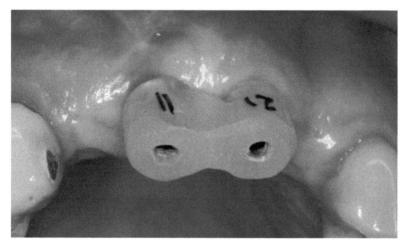

Figure 5.23 Locating jig for case 5.16 showing position of the abutments.

● Given information about the treatment they have completed which should include:
  - the type of implants
  - details of the surgical procedure including any augmentation
  - details of the prosthesis (screw or cement retained)
  - the type of abutment
  - the maintenance care regime and follow-up care
  - the baseline probing chart and radiographs taken after the fit of the prosthesis

Outcomes:

The different approaches and timelines used for delivering implant-retained restorations should take into consideration the pretreatment planning during which decisions about the type of prosthesis, the anticipated timing of restoration and loading will have been considered. However, the most predictable outcomes have been seen largely with the conventional way of implant placement and restoration with delayed placement and conventional loading being the most favoured option today. The former approach should always be the option of choice when there are patient-related risk factors and site-related factors that may compromise the treatment outcome irrespective of the reported success rates ranging from 96% to 98% across all methods. If predictability is to be achieved, then planning for the type of restoration, when it is to be delivered and loaded should be undertaken at the outset when the start of the plan is being considered as these decisions will drive the surgical placement.

Key Learning Points

- Describe the process involved in surgical placement of implants
- Discuss the factors that affect surgical placement of implants
- Consider the importance of the sequential site preparation and primary stability when placing implants
- Explain the rationale and principles for augmentation and understand the applications
- Describe the materials used for augmentation
- Explain the types of implant-retained prosthesis and the differences and roles
- Consider the key stages of constructing an implant-retained prosthesis
- Identify the challenges with occlusal form on success
- Show an awareness of the minor and major complications associated with implant-retained prosthesis
- Demonstrate an understanding of the role of prosthetic design and form on long-term outcome of implant treatment

References

1 Mericske-Stern, R. (2008). Prosthetic considerations. *Australian Dental Journal* 53 (1): S49–59.
2 Boyce, R. (2021). Prosthodontic principles in dental implantology. *Dental Clinics of North America* 65 (1): 135–165.

6

Peri-Implant Tissues

The peri-implant tissues are the tissues that surround the osseointegrated implants and are divided into the soft and hard tissue compartments. The soft tissue compartment, known as the peri-implant mucosa, is the tissue being referred to when the term 'peri-implant tissues' is used. This tissue is formed during the healing process that follows once implant placement and healing abutment connection has been completed for two-piece implants and following implant placement when a one-piece implant is placed. This soft tissue implant interface plays an important role as it forms a biological seal around the implant providing protection against the oral surrounding. The seal also isolates the implant and bone from the oral environment through an attachment which limits the ingrowth of bacterial plaque thereby preventing disease at this interface.

Whilst the concept of osseointegration is widely accepted, as the demand for implant treatment increases, an understanding of this soft tissue seal, its role and the factors that can affect it are essential to ensure the long-term stability of the tissues and the implant restoration and its successful outcome. A number of factors will influence the stability of this seal and include the degree of keratinised tissue present, the abutment materials and surface topography of the implant. Some of these factors will be identified at the outset during the early planning stages and knowing these will help plan a regime directed at reducing their impact. Thus, pretreatment planning is not only important for the provision of the prosthesis but is also critical to help ensure that factors that could place the future stability of the peri-implant tissues at risk are identified and managed as early as possible and the patient made aware of their implications.

Anatomy:

An understanding of the similarities and differences between the tooth–soft tissue interface and the peri-implant soft tissue will also help provide a clearer recognition of deviations from health and the possible reasons (Table 6.1). The main differences between these two interfaces lie in the following areas:

● Junctional Epithelial Component

Both teeth and implants have a long junctional epithelium which is also known as the barrier epithelium. Around implants, this is thinner and longer and has a hemidesmosomal attachment with the transmucosal abutment and a thin basal layer. This feature

Dental Implants for Hygienists and Therapists, First Edition. Ulpee Darbar.
© 2022 John Wiley & Sons Ltd. Published 2022 by John Wiley & Sons Ltd.

Table 6.1 Similarities and Differences between the Tissues around Teeth and the Peri-Implant Tissue.

Features	Tissues around Teeth	Peri-Implant Tissues
Gingival sulcus depth	Shallow on average around 2–3 mm	Variable and is dependent on the depth at which the implant is placed and the abutment length and restoration margin
Junctional epithelium	Hemidesmosome attachment to enamel	Hemidesmosome attachment to titanium
Gingival fibres	Complex array of fibres inserting into the cementum about the crestal bone and onto the periosteum	No fibre insertion into the implant; fibres are oriented parallel, or circumferential to the long axis of the implant
Connective tissue attachment	Well-organised collagen fibre bundles running perpendicular to the root cementum	Structure that is rich in collagen but no fibroblasts and vascularity
Blood supply	Numerous vascular anastomoses between the vessels from the periodontal ligament space, and gingival connective tissue	Fewer blood vessels and majority of the supply coming from the underlying periosteum
Biologic width	Junctional epithelium – 0.97 mm; CTA – 1.07 mm	JE = 1.88 mm and CT = 1.05 mm

along with the collagen fibre orientation increases the risk of bacterial penetration around the implant (Figure 6.1a, b).

- Connective Tissue Component

There is a higher fibre content around implants with a lower cellular content and the collagen fibres are arranged parallel to the implant surface with fewer fibroblasts in contrast to teeth where the fibres are perpendicular. As a result, when assessing the peri-implant tissues with a probe, a deeper depth will be noted when compared to teeth and the mean bleeding on probing

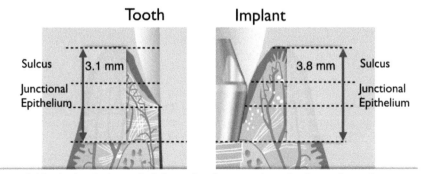

1. Vertical soft tissue height on implants and teeth, drawn based on the data by Berglundh et al (1)

Figure 6.1 Shows the anatomy of the tissues around teeth and dental implants.

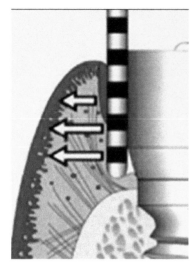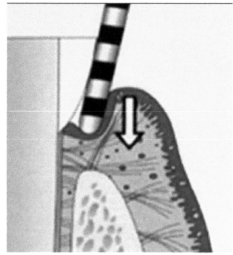

Figure 6.2 Probing around implants vs teeth (reproduced from intecopen - kripal & Chandrasekaran).

is also much higher. The delicate nature of the tissue also makes this area more sensitive to pressure and increase in probing pressure/force may lead to trauma to the tissues (Figure 6.2).

● Vascularity

The vascularity around implants comes from the periosteum of the bone with few to no blood vessels in the zone adjacent to the implant surface. This reduced vascularity affects the healing by reducing the number of circulating neutrophils and B cells in the area.

● Periodontal Ligament

Implants lack a periodontal ligament and thus when disease or injury due to occlusal trauma takes place, the effects are transmitted to the bone directly.

● Healing Response of the Tissues

The cellular response around teeth and implants is different as the sites around implants are infiltrated with B cells and plasma cells. Due to this, and the lack of a tight supracrestal connective tissue compartment, disease progression is much more rapid around peri-implant tissues. The number of circulating neutrophils and B cells is also reduced due to the reduced vascular blood supply.

● Biologic Width

This width varies around implants and is dependant on the depth of the implant placement. It ranges upto 3 mm (1–1.8 mm junctional epithelium and 1–2 mm connective tissue attachment). When the width is reduced, marginal bone resorption will take place. Factors that may influence its dimensions are the type of implant (one vs two piece), implant material (titanium, gold alloy, zirconium) implant surface characteristics (surface topography, macrodesign), loading protocol and the flap design used for implant placement. Whilst it is thought that these factors will affect the biologic width, the degree to which this happens remains unclear (Figure 6.3a, b).

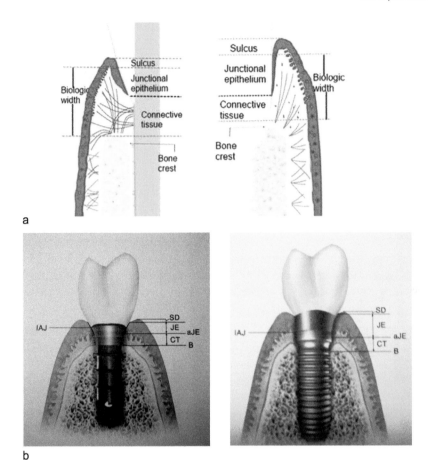

Figure 6.3 a: Biologic width around implants. b: Difference between one-piece (tissue level) and one-piece (bone level) implants.

Periimplant tissues in Health

The health of the peri-implant tissues is essential for long-term stability and should be monitored throughout the planned treatment after implant placement.

Figure 6.4 shows the tissues around a two-piece implant when the healing abutment has been removed. The shape of the tissues has been characterised by the use of a shaped healing abutment for the optimal emergence profile of the prosthesis.

The tight gingival cuff has the same protective function as around teeth and is made up of epithelium and connective tissue which forms during the post-surgical healing period after implant placement. It is thought that with two-piece implant systems, the repeated removal of the healing abutment, leads to the hemidesmosomal attachment being traumatised thus leading to the instability of the gingival margin which can become an issue around implants with thin quality tissue biotype. The benefits of keratinised tissue around dental implants have been discussed previously. The peri-implant soft tissue that forms is described as 'scar tissue' which has impaired resistance to bacterial colonisation and the biological seal formed even in healthy tissues is weak and has poor mechanical resistance. When this seal is disturbed, the health of

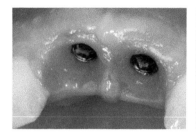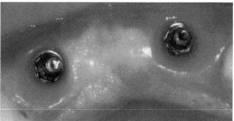

Figure 6.4 Peri-implant soft tissues after removal of the healing abutment. The health of the tissue is evident; however, the redness is caused by the breaking of the hemidesmosomal attachment when the abutment is removed.

the tissue is compromised leading to disease and ultimately implant failure. The patient's daily plaque control does play a key role in maintaining the health of the peri-implant tissues.

Healthy peri-implant tissues will have an absence of clinical signs of inflammation (redness and swelling), no bleeding on probing and probing depths < 5 mm although this depth will vary with the depth of the implant fixture placement. The following steps should be followed to detect if the peri-implant tissues are healthy:

- Visual inspection of the tissues which should show no signs of disease.
- Probing pocket depths may vary depending on the depth of implant placement; however, an increase in depth compared to baseline indicates presence of disease.
- Lack of bleeding on probing should be assessed with light forces to minimise the risk of trauma to the tissues.
- Absence of further bone loss > 2 mm measured against the baseline radiographs.

Peri-Implant Tissues: Disease

The prevalence of peri-implant disease is increasing as the demand for implant treatment rises. The early identification of inflammation will help implement prompt and effective intervention which will assist in achieving health. However, the outcome will be dependent on the reasons for the inflammation. The standard checks listed above should be undertaken at every visit to ensure that early signs of disease are not missed.

- Factors to Consider:

The factors that increase the risk of peri-implant disease include (Figure 6.5):

- Patient related:

Ability to maintain an optimal level of plaque control with effective home care regimes; smoking; uncontrolled diabetes, history of periodontitis.

- Prosthesis related:

The design of the prosthesis, its shape and contour will be key to ensuring that the patient can clean around the prosthesis. A poorly designed prosthesis will impede cleaning leading to a higher risk of inflammation and disease.

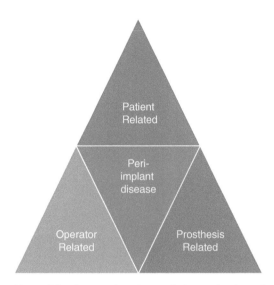

Figure 6.5 Factors that play a role in peri-implant disease manifestation.

- Operator related:

Placement of the implants and their proximity to teeth and each other as well as designing the prosthesis.

Peri-implant diseases have been related to biological and mechanical factors. The former relies on the concept of these conditions being infections and are described using the presence of bleeding, changes in the crestal bone levels and deepening of peri-implant pockets. Mechanical factors are related to the unfavourable stresses that can be generated as a result of occlusal trauma leading to marginal bone loss. Bacterial biofilms made of bacteria and saliva colonize the implant surface and have been noted to be responsible for 65% of peri-implant diseases. The daily chemomechanical removal and disruption of this biofilm will reduce the risk of disease. In the partially dentate patient, the migration of bacteria from the teeth to the implants is well known. If not removed efficiently, an inflammatory response is elicited which releases cytokines which enhance the collection of neutrophils. If treatment is implemented at this stage, then the condition will reverse itself; however, if the bacteria continue to persist, then more neutrophils infiltrate the tissues leading to further destruction, with the host response to the inflammation leading to bone loss around the implants. As the situation continues to progress, increased infiltrates of proinflammatory cells responsible for further tissue breakdown is seen with eventual loss of the implant itself. The bacteria that have been implicated in peri-implant disease belong to the group of campylocbacters, aggregatibacter actinomycetum comitans and trepenomena.

- Peri-implant diseases

The two most common peri-implant diseases that have been reported are:

- Periimplant mucositis (Figure 6.6)
  - Defined as the presence of signs of inflammation noted as redness, swelling, line or drop of bleeding within 30 s following probing with no additional bone loss following initial healing. It is reported to resemble gingivitis.

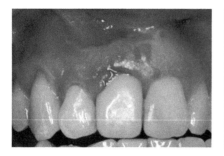
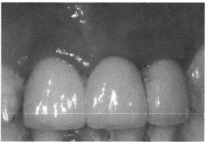
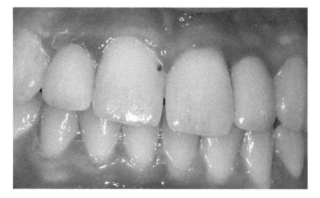

Figure 6.6 Peri-implant mucositis.

- – Reversible condition.
- – Prevalence reported at 30–62.6% at implant level and 47–80% at patient level.
- – Aetiology is poor oral hygiene and compliance to advice, poor prosthesis design, poor fit of the prosthesis, poor position of implants, lack of keratinised mucosa and retained cement, rarely titanium alloy hypersensitivity.
- – Clinical signs: bleeding on probing with or without suppuration.
- – Progression will lead to peri-implantitis.

● Peri-implantitis (Figure 6.7)

- – Defined as an inflammatory reaction associated with the loss of supporting bone beyond the initial biologic remodelling around an implant in function. Reported to resemble periodontitis and has similar microbial flora and gram negative anaerobes.
- – Irreversible condition.
- – Prevalence rate of 12–43% at implant sites and 28–56% of patient level.
- – Aetiology combination of bacteria or stress or both.
- – Clinical signs: bleeding, increased pocket depths, recession, crater-like osseous defects localised around the implant, mucosal swelling and erythema, absence of pain; radiographic evidence of bone loss.
- – Progression will lead to implant loss.

Patients with a history of periodontitis have a higher risk of peri-implantitis with reduced survival rates. Smoking and the use of tobacco also causes a higher risk of complications and peri-implant disease. Patients who had a history of periodontitis and smoking have

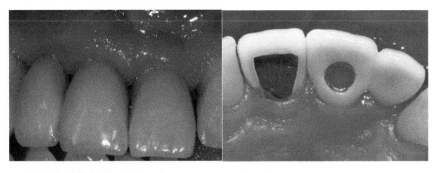

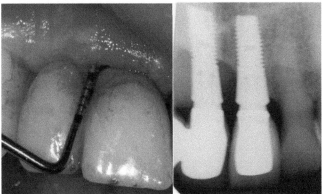

Figure 6.7   Peri-implantitis.

been shown to have a higher risk of peri-implant disease. Occlusal stresses caused by unfavourable loads due to parafunction can initiate bone loss further compounded by bacterial loads thus increasing the risk of peri-implantitis. It has also been suggested that the acidic environment caused by the bacteria can lead to the release of titanium ions from the surface of the implant generating a local inflammatory response. Poorly controlled diabetes will increase the risk of peri-implantitis. Keratinised mucosa affects the long-term health of the peri-implant tissues and will provide patient comfort and ease of plaque removal. Peri-implantitis progresses in a non-linear accelerating pattern and for the majority of cases the onset tends to be within three years of function.

Classification systems have been proposed for distinguishing different degrees of severity of peri-implant disease. The Froum and Rosen classification was based on the probing depths and bone loss with the disease being divided into three clinical stages and that proposed by Schwarz et al., which classified the defects, is based on the figuration of the intrabony component. Spikermann et al. used a five-category characterisation of the peri-implant defect and others used the amount of bone loss. The classification that is currently recommended was proposed by the consensus workshop and includes grading and staging of the disease as shown in Table 6.2.

Irrespective of the biological factors related to peri-implant diseases, one of the main contributory factors contributory to peri-implant disease is the incorrect placement of dental implants and poorly contoured restorations impeding plaque control. These implants are placed in either unacceptable or unfavourable positions and cause localised disease due to poor access leading to plaque accumulation and or lack of bone (Figure 6.8a, b).

Table 6.2 Different Classification Systems Used for Peri-Implantitis.

Classification	Types	Characteristics
Froum and Rosen (2012)	Early	Probing depths ≥ 4 mm (bleeding &/or suppuration on probing Bone loss <25% of the implant length
	Moderate	Probing depths ≥ 6 mm (bleeding &/or suppuration on probing) Bone loss 25–50% of implant length
	Advanced	Probing Depth ≥ 8 mm (bleeding &/or suppuration on probing) Bone loss > 50% of implant length
Schwartz et al. (2007)	Class 1	a = combined horizontal and vertical loss of the adjacent vestibular alveolar bone
		b = higher dehiscence values than Class Ia defects and identifiable by mesial and distal
		c = additional circumferential components
		d = clear mesial and distal component with oral and vestibular dehiscence
		E = clear mesial, distal, vestibular and oral component without dehiscence
	Class II	Consistent horizontal bone loss, identifiable as supraalveolar exposition of the implant
Spikermann et al. (1984)	Class I	Horizontal
	Class II	Hey shaped
	Class III a	Funnel shaped
	Class III b	Gap like
	Class IV	Horizontal circular
Nashimura et al. (1997)	Class 1	Slight horizontal bone loss with minimal peri-implant defects
	Class 2	Moderate horizontal bone loss with isolated vertical defects
	Class 3	Moderate to advanced horizontal bone loss with broad, circular bony defects
	Class 4	Advanced horizontal bone loss with broad, circumferential vertical defects, as well as loss of the oral and/or vestibular bony wall
Berglundh et al. (2018)	Peri-implant health	Absence of visual signs of inflammation and bleeding on probing Can exist around implants with normal or reduced bone Not possible to define a range of probing depths
	Peri-implant mucositis	Visual signs of inflammation and bleeding on probing
	Peri-implantitis	Inflammation of the peri-implant mucosa Progressive loss of supporting bone
	Peri-implant soft and hard tissue deficiencies	Deficiencies preoperatively following tooth extraction in implant placement sites

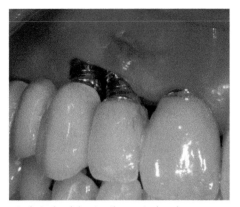

a: Implants placed close together causing bone loss

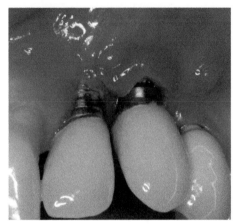

b: Buccally placed implants causing inflammation, pocketing and bone loss

Figure 6.8   a, b: Incorrect implant position leading to peri-implantitis.

Peri-implant Tissue: Assessment

The tissues should be assessed carefully and the details of the steps that need to be followed are given in the next chapter. The main focus when assessing the peri-implant tissues is to establish the presence of inflammation and should include a visual examination and a probing examination. Both of these will help establish the health of the peri-implant tissues.

Peri-Implant Disease: Treatment

Treatment is essential if the disease is to be managed effectively. However, there is no standard consensus on how to treat peri-implant disease. Different protocols have been advocated, and these aim at controlling the bacterial biofilm and correcting the underlying bone defect. The most important aspect of managing peri-implant disease is to ensure that the home care is at an optimal standard and a revision of the oral hygiene techniques used should be undertaken. Details of this are covered in the next chapter. The value of excellent home care regime cannot be underestimated, and there is a direct correlation between poor oral hygiene and peri-implant bone loss.

● Non-surgical treatment

This is successful for peri-implant mucositis and with good patient compliance resolves the issue. However, the outcome for peri-implantitis is variable and is most likely related to the challenge of removing the biofilm from the contaminated implant threads.

– When managing peri-implantitis non-surgically, the aim is to use instrumentation, hand or mechanically driven, to disrupt the biofilm. Adjuncts, such as topical antibiotics can be used to detoxify the implant surface and provide a local concentration of antibacterial agent in the pocket (Figure 6.10a, b). Systemic antibiotics can also be used; however, unless there is systemic involvement the use of these should be limited to minimise the risk of antibiotic resistance. Amino acid glycine powder has also been used with air polishers due to its low abrasivity. It is effective at removing biofilm without damaging the soft tissues or the implant. A post-treatment rinse should

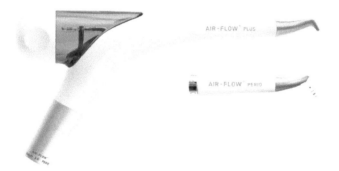

Figure 6.9 Air polisher: these use kinetic energy in the flow of aerated water with a powder (usually bicarbonate based, amino acid glycines and some have used plant-based sugars) to remove the biofilm from the surface. For use around implants special tips that can be inserted into the subgingival area need to be used as seen in the picture. The site must be rinsed of all residual powder.

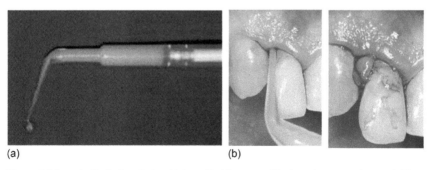

(a)   (b)

Figure 6.10   a, b: Topical antimicrobial applied into a residual pocket around a tooth. The same principles apply around implants.

be used to remove any residue (Figure 6.9).Ultrasonic instrumentation can be used with the dedicated plastic tips the details of which are covered in the next chapter.

- Lasers have also been advocated for treating peri-implantitis and include the diode laser, Nd-YAG, erbium or carbon dioxide. The effectiveness remains debatable with mixed information about their effectiveness when compared to conventional forms of treatment. The following approaches have been used:

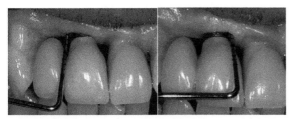

a: Improvement in the inflammation after non surgical debridement but residual pocketing

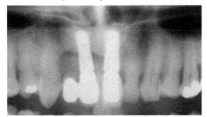

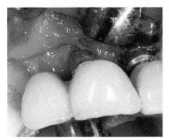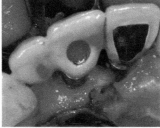

b: Resective Surgery to Reduce the pocket: Full thickness flap is raised; the bone defect identified bone reshaped and flap closed apically.

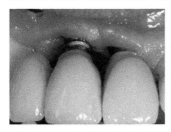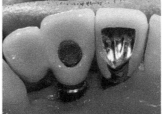

c: Post surgery healing showing the tissue shrinkage and exposure of the implant threads.

Figure 6.11A   Resective surgical management of peri-implantitis.

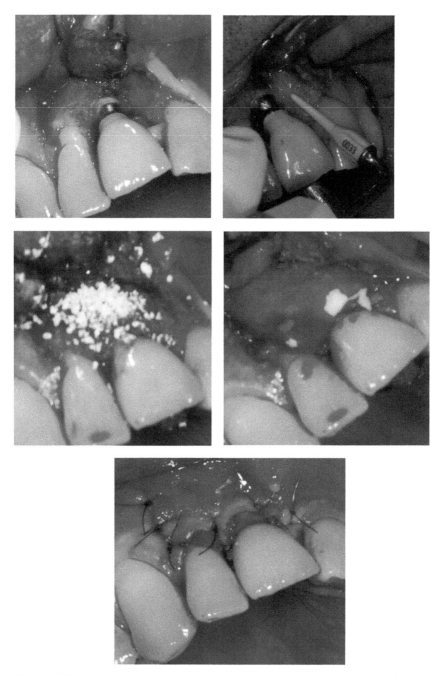

Figure 6.11B Regenerative surgical management of peri-implantitis. Flap raised in a patient with persistent probing depths; flap is raised and the site is debrided using special piezo tip for implants. The mesial defect is identified and the site grafted using cow bone and a pig-based barrier and the flap replaced and stabilised with stitches.

During non-surgical therapy, the laser beam is directed at the inflamed soft tissue in the sulcus and aims to disrupt the biofilm and decontaminate the pocket. For surgical procedures, the laser is used to remove the diseased epithelial lining and in some cases they are used to raise the flap and decontaminate the site and undertake osseous recontouring.

– Photodynamic therapy

The laser light activates a photosensitizer that has been placed into the pocket and provides an antimicrobial effect.

– Photobiomodulation

This is a non-thermal technique which elicits photophysical and photochemical events and is used to promote wound healing and tissue regeneration.

– Surgical Treatment

Whilst non-surgical therapy will provide a positive outcome, in peri-implantitis patients, due to the underlying bone defect, surgical intervention is inevitably needed to gain access to the site, to disinfect the contaminated implant surface accepting that re-osseointegration will not take place as the surface is contaminated and correct the underlying bone defect. The approach used to manage the latter is dependent on the anatomy of the defect and whether the bone defect has a crater, an intrabony component or is horizontal it will involve regeneration or reshaping the defect to apically reposition the flap. The surgical treatment will commence with a flap and exposure of the defect followed by thorough debridement and removal of all granulation tissue. The use of titanium brushes have been advocated; however, small particles of the brush have been found in sites afterwards. Air polishing with powder can also be used. Alongside the mechanical debridement, chemical decontamination has also been suggested with citric acid or doxycycline. If the defect shape is horizontal then osseous recontouring is undertaken before the flap is replaced and sutured. In sites with crater defects or intrabony defects, augmentation/regeneration can be undertaken using one of the materials described in Chapter 5. Figures 6.11a, b show the surgical procedures used to manage peri-implantitis. There are specific parameters that need to be observed when considering regeneration around these sites and they include:

- Prosthesis must be checked and the need for recontouring considered.
- The occlusion must be checked to ensure that there is no overload.
- Establish the number of bone walls remaining.

Other materials that have been suggested for use are enamel matrix-derived proteins. The correction of the contours prosthesis are an integral part of the surgical management as failure to do so when the prosthetic shape compromises cleaning will lead to recurrence of the problems and implant failure.

Surgical treatment is also needed when there is lack of keratinised tissue, thin gingival tissue biotype or both. In these situations, the non-surgical protocol should be followed and a decision about the need for and type of soft tissue graft made and undertaken depending on the objective. Lack of keratinised tissue will necessitate a free gingival graft (Figure 6.12a, b, c).

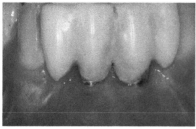
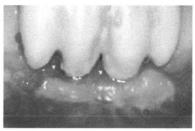

a: Lack of keratinised tissue causing recurring infections; Post free gingival graft symptoms resolved completely

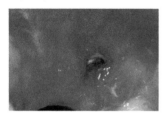
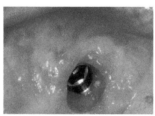

b: Lack of keratinsied tissue around implant; Free gingival graft used to enhance tissue prior to reconstruction

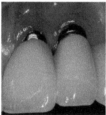
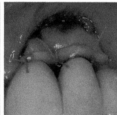
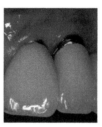

c: Connective Tissue Graft with epithelial collar used to enhance tissue volume and increase keratinised tissue

Figure 6.12   a, b, c: Compromised gingival tissues around implants showing the use of different soft tissue grafts to improve the gingival tissue health.

Protocols for managing peri-implantitis have been advocated following a systematic pathway and includes the Cumulative Interceptive Supportive Therapy (CIST) protocol which incorporates the clinical signs of disease into the protocol (Figure 6.13).

The different treatment modalities for peri-implant diseases are shown in figure 6.14 and summarised in Table 6.3.

Key Learning Points

- Describe the peri-implant soft tissue interface and the differences compared to a tooth.
- Discuss the assessment parameters to be used when assessing peri-implant tissues.
- Explain the risk factors increasing the risk of peri-implant disease.
- Describe the different peri-implant disease types and their diagnosis.
- Consider the management options for peri-implant diseases.
- Describe the treatment options and protocols for both peri-implant mucositis and peri-implantitis

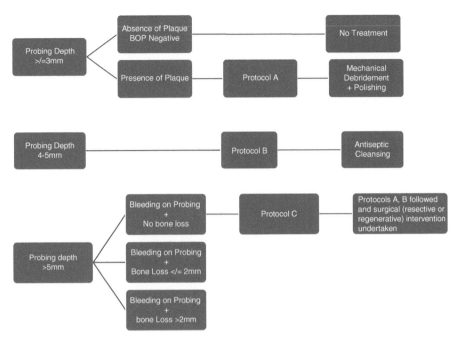

Figure 6.13 Cumulative interceptive supportive therapy (CIST) of peri-implant mucositis and peri-implantitis.

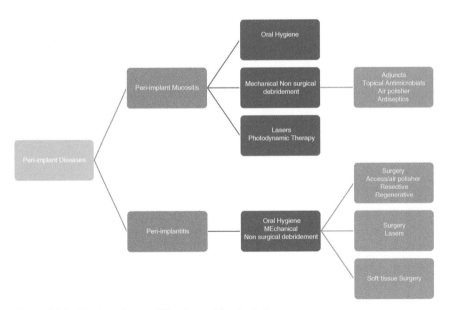

Figure 6.14 Treatment modalities for peri-implant disease.

Table 6.3 Treatment Modalities for Peri-Implant Disease: The hygienist plays a strategic role in the monitoring, assessment and initial management.

Assessment of Peri-Implant Tissues

Essential and crucial to establish the presence of disease and should be undertaken at two levels:

1. Tissue and Bone assessment: Visually and using a probe as well as radiographs. Probing is critical to identify the early signs of disease with bleeding, and the tissues should be assessed visually, and clinically with the probing depths measured against those recorded after the fit of the prosthesis. The loss of bone should be interpreted carefully and measured against the bone levels at the time of fitting the prosthesis.

2. Position of the implants and prosthetic contours: These should also be assessed as often they be the contributory/exacerbating factors. If the position and contours are inadequate then management should include addressing these parameters as well.

3. **Patient made aware of the risks and the challenge and involved in the decision making of the next steps.**

Type of Peri-Implant Disease	Steps to follow	Considerations
Peri-Implant Mucositis *Reversible* inflammatory reaction in the soft tissue surrounding an implant. Characterised by: • Visual signs of inflammation • Bleeding on probing • Swelling of the peri-implant tissues • Pain and discomfort • Increased probing depths (usually false) *Desired Treatment Outcome:* *Reduction in Bleeding and Probing Depths*	A. Plaque control and oral hygiene measures	Manual, electric brushes; interdental brushes (tepes, single tufted; superfloss) water flossers/picks; Smoking cessation advice and control of risk factors
	B. Adjunctive non-surgical debridement With or without locally applied adjuncts (e.g. antimicrobials/chemotherapeutics)	Use resin/fibre or titanium currettes; Ultrasonic scalers with special inserts or rubber tips; Other techniques: Photodynamic therapy, lasers, mixed outcomes
	C. Address any restorative factors compromising access for cleaning	Liaise with the dentist; remove the prosthesis and reshape to allow access for cleaning
	D. Surgery: usually where there is gingival tissue excess and overgrowth	Tends to be resective soft tissue surgery either as a gingivectomy or flap. Should not be undertaken until B, C have been completed

Peri-implantitis		
Irreversible inflammatory reaction with bone loss; usually has deepening probing depths and recession around implants Characterised by: ● Visual signs of inflammation which may include swelling ● Bleeding on probing ± suppuration ● Increasing probing depths ● Progressive loss of crestal supporting bone	Follow Steps A, B, C first and reassess The occlusion should be assessed and any parafunctional activity evaluated Depending on the type of prosthesis this may need to be looked at carefully	If the key issue relates to the position of the implants and the poor contour of the prosthesis then explantation may be the desired outcome If there is an occlusal problem, this needs to be addressed as part of the initial management
	D, Resective surgery with or without bone recontouring	This is dependant on the nature of the bone loss. If there are no crater or intrabony defects, then reshaping of the bone with apical reposition of the flap should be considered; Implant surface cleansing – no clear evidence that this will work
Desired Outcome *Reduction in bleeding and pocket depth reduction and stabilisation of the bone loss* *Prolong the life of the implant*	E. Regenerative Surgery	Usually if there is a crater/intrabony defect. The focus is to fill the defect as re-osseintegration will not happen as the implant surface is contaminated
	F. Soft tissue surgery	Lack of keratinised tissue and thin biotype; then a free gingival graft or a connective tissue graft may need to be considered if there are no other probing depths or issues.
	G. Explantation	Poor implant position, poor prosthetic contours and poor access; consider augmentation at the time of explantation to maintain the bone quantity.

Follow up and monitoring with adjunctive maintenance care are crucial to maintain status quo but patient should be warned of the poor long-term compromise and outcome

References

1 Thakur, R., Gaur, V., Yadav, B., and Venkitram, N. (2020). Biology of Peri-implant tissues: A review. *Journal of Dental and Medical Sciences* 19: 18–24.

2 Winstein, T., Clauser, T., Del Fabbor, M., Deflorian, A., Taschieri, S., Testorie, T., and Francetti, L. (2020). Prevalence of peri-implantitis: A mulitcentred cross sectional study on 248 patients. *Journal of Dentistry* 8: 80.

3 Revert, S., Turger Persson, G., Fq, P., and Pm, C. (2018). Peri-implant health, peri-implant mucositis and peri-implantitis: Case definition and diagnostic considerations. *Journal of Clinical Periodontology* 45 (supl 20): 5278–5285.

4 Wang, Y., Zhang, Y., and Miron, R. (2015). Health, maintenance and recovery of soft tissues around implants. *Clinical Implant Dentistry and Related Research* 18 (3).

5 Valente, N.A. and Andreaana, S. (2016). Peri-implant disease: What we know and what we need to know. *Journal of Periodontal & Implant Science* 46 (3): 135051.

6 Hashim, D., Cionca, N., Combescure, C., and Mombelli, A. (2018). The diagnosis of peri-implantitis: A Systematic Review on the predictive value of bleeding on probing. *Clinical Oral Implants Research* 29 (suppl 16): 276–293.

7 Pssi, D., Singh, M., Dutta, S.R., Sharma, S., Atri, M., Ahlawat, J., and Jain, A. (2017). Newer proposed classification of peri-implant defects: A critical update. *Journal of Oral Biology and Craniofacial Research* 7 (1): 58–61.

8 Mombelli, A. and Lang, N.P. (1998). The diagnosis and treatment of peri-implantitis. *Periodontology* 17: 63–76.

9 Schwarz, F., Derks, J., Monje, A., and Hl, W. (2018). Peri-**implantitis**. *Journal of Clinical Periodontology* 45 (Suppl 20 Jun): S246–S266.

7

Maintenance Care around Dental Implants

The long-term success of dental implant restorations is dependent on customised and focussed follow-up protocols taking into consideration the risk predictors that may influence the outcome using a team approach. A risk predictor is any factor that may influence and increase the chances of the disease occurring. The proposed maintenance regime should be considered when the implant treatment is planned and should take into consideration the risk factors that are established during the generic and site-specific planning phases. The patients' journey through this planned pathway will help to establish the risk predictors that will need to be taken into account when planning the maintenance regime. This early consideration will foster a preventive approach with careful case selection, pre-operative patient education and risk assessment to manage and control the identified risk factors and predictors implicated in the increased risk of both biological and technical implant-related complications covered in previous chapters. The approach will help identify patients at risk of these complications especially peri-implant disease at the outset and the patient engaged into the discussion prior to any intervention being started. Concerns with patient compliance should be taken into consideration before any implant treatment is executed until the patient understands and accepts responsibility for the aftercare following completion of the treatment. The need for stringent maintenance protocols for the 'at risk' patient is even more important and is driven by the differences between implants and teeth where the latter are more resistant to disease progression unlike implants where disease progression is often rapid due to the lack of the periodontal ligament and variation in the vascularity.

Definition

Maintenance care, also known as supportive therapy, is defined as the continuous care initiated after the completion of active treatment at regular intervals aimed at ensuring that the health of the tissues is monitored and maintained, and deviation from health identified early so that timely intervention can be implemented to minimise the risk of the problem worsening (Figure 7.1). The problems around implants will fall into two categories, those related to technical issues and those related to biological issues, both of which have been previously discussed (see Chapter 6). The key aims of a maintenance visit are to:

Dental Implants for Hygienists and Therapists, First Edition. Ulpee Darbar.
© 2022 John Wiley & Sons Ltd. Published 2022 by John Wiley & Sons Ltd.

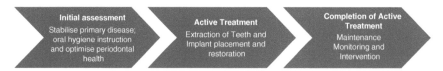

Figure 7.1

- Monitor the tissues around the implants (visual and clinical assessment)
- Identify problems early and intervene as necessary

The visit is crucial to carry out timely intervention which helps minimise the risk of disease progression as failure to implement treatment is likely to result in progressive and rapid bone loss with ultimate implant loss. Patients should be monitored at customised time intervals based on their risk profile and ideally each visit should include an assessment of:

- The patients plaque control
- The peri-implant tissues and their status
- The implant-retained prosthesis

Principles

The key principles of a maintenance visit are checking the above and executing treatment to maintain and/or manage issues that have been identified. The monitoring should be more stringent during the first year and should be undertaken at least once every 3–4 months, and if the situation remains stable, this can be tailored to longer intervals depending on patient compliance, risk profile and manual dexterity. The assessment undertaken during maintenance should be evaluated against the baseline information recorded following the fit of the prosthesis which is crucial in helping explain future change. It is important to remember that the care provided should be continuous, individualised and undertaken systematically. In order to monitor the disease, an understanding of the signs of disease, the type of implant system and treatment undertaken along with the type of prosthesis and materials used at the soft tissue interface is important. An awareness of the implant soft tissue interface will assist with ensuring confidence when undertaking the maintenance visits. The patient should, ideally, have been given 'an end of treatment passport' which contains the following information:

- The teeth being replaced
- The implant system (one piece or two piece)
- The details of implant surgery (date, type, timing, augmentation)
- The details of the prosthesis (date of fit, type – screw retained or cement, type of abutments used, one piece or two piece, the loading protocol used)
- The type of cement used (if cement retained) and if screw retained, the type of driver
- The baseline probing chart and radiograph following the fit of the prosthesis including date recorded
- The risk profile of the patient and specific concerns

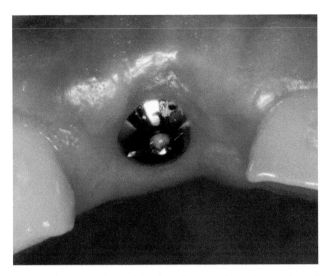

Figure 7.2a: Healthy peri-implant tissues prior to impression taking.

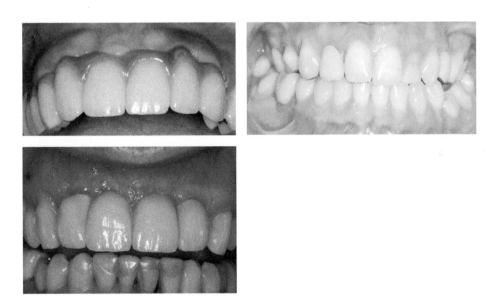

Figure 7.2b: Healthy peri-implant tissues around implants that have been in situ for > five years. The patients are on regular maintenance programme. Patient with a upper fixed reconstruction; patient with a single tooth replacing UL 4 showing health tissues; patient with a 15-year-old implant-retained bridge anteriorly with healthy tissues

- The recommended maintenance regime
- Any other issues of note

Healthy peri-implant tissues should show no redness or inflammation (Figure 7.2a, b), and if bleeding is noted, then this is a sign of early disease. The clinical assessment is multifaceted and includes the patient-related assessment and the clinical assessment. Insufficient clinical skills related to the assessment, planning and judging the design of the prosthesis and ability to recognise key patient-related factors such as parafunction (bruxism), smoking, uncontrolled diabetes and periodontal disease are significant contributory factors towards implant failure. The latter conditions predispose the patient to a greater risk of complications and failure and thus early identification will help mitigate this risk.

Components of Maintenance Care

A typical maintenance care visit should include the following:

Patient Assessment

- Presenting complaint
  The patient's awareness of any issues should be established. Patients are astute and very aware of what is going on in their mouth and will usually be able to describe changes they have noticed early. It is important that these concerns are heard and relevant measures taken to address them. Specific questions related to the patients awareness of bleeding, looseness or movement of the prosthesis should be asked. Patients may present within the first six months of their prosthesis being fitted complaining of loose crowns. This is usually related to occlusal loading driven by the lack of proprioception around implants which enables the patient to place loads of up to 100 Newtons around implants without realising this. This differential loading can lead to loosening of the crown, and if cemented, the crown will come off and if screw retained, then the screw will come loose. This can also be seen as a late complication in patients with old implant restorations that have been in place for more than five years and as the wear of the natural teeth occurs over time, the implant-retained prosthesis is left in occlusal overload leading to the looseness.

- Update of the medical history and social history
  The medical history may change during the course of the follow-up period and should be updated at each visit. Conditions such as late onset diabetes could change within a short period of time, which if uncontrolled, could affect the outcome of the implant treatment, and reduced salivary flow either due to aging or medications can also affect the bacterial biofilms and healing of the mucosal tissues. Other conditions such as oral mucosal disorders which cause soreness of the gingival tissues may affect the patients ability to brush around the area and autoimmune conditions such as rheumatoid arthritis which can affect manual dexterity compromising the daily cleaning can also have a detrimental effect on the health of the tissues around implants. The hormonal changes due to pregnancy have been shown to influence the situation in the mouth and can affect peri-implant tissues. The prevalence of conditions such as dementia is on the rise, and it is important to remember that patients with early and undiagnosed dementia may present during this phase and the need for early recognition is important. The patients' smoking and vaping history should also be checked.

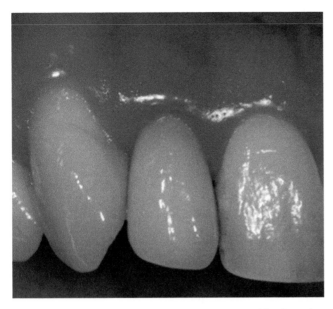

Figure 7.3 Early signs of peri-implant disease noted by the redness and loss of stippling of the gingival tissues around the UR 2 implant.

Clinical Assessment

- Soft tissues:
  A visual assessment should be undertaken of the tissues and signs of inflammation (redness, swelling, loss of stippling and sinus tracts) noted. The tissues around implants should be assessed. Any signs of redness will indicate a possible inflammatory lesion (Figure 7.3). Sites with lack of keratinised tissue and mobile mucosal tissue will need to be assessed carefully as these areas will have a tendency to harbour bacteria. These sites are usually associated with bone loss and increased plaque accumulation with recession and inflammation and a higher frequency of bleeding due to the lack of the supracrestal hemidesmosomal attachment (Figure 7.4). The gingival tissue biotype should also be noted especially around the implants with thin biotype usually being associated with lack of keratinised tissue and increased risk of recession. Keratinised gingival tissue provides improved long-term stability and is more resistant to abrasion and enables ease of cleaning.

- Plaque and bleeding indices
  This should be assessed at individual sites and also across the whole mouth. The plaque index should be recorded and the indices recommended for use around implants are shown in Table 7.1. Plaque in the site is detected by gently running the probe over the margins around the implant tissue interface and also on the implant and the prosthetic surface. Despite early belief stating that rough surface implants harbour subgingival bacteria and colonisation is influenced by the implant thus contributing to a higher risk of peri-implant disease, there is no evidence to support this belief. Bleeding on probing is a better indicator of the presence of inflammation however, around implants, the nature

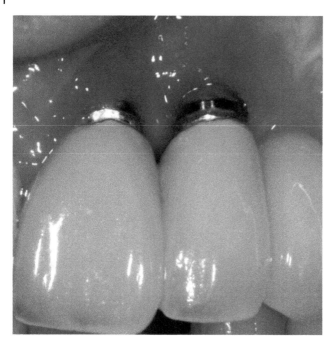

Figure 7.4 Shows the presence of gingival recession and inflammation around the UL 1, 2 implants where there is thin gingival tissue biotype and lack of keratinised gingival tissue.

Table 7.1 Plaque Indices Used for Plaque Assessment around Peri-Implant Tissues.

Group	Indicated for	Scoring	Comments
O'Leary et al.	Mainly teeth but can be used around implants	% score	Calculated using number of tooth surfaced with plaque divided by the number of tooth surfaces present × 100
Lindquist et al.	Mainly for implants	0, 1, 2	0 = no visible plaque 1 = local plaque accumulation 2 = general plaque accumulation > 25%
Mombelli et al.	Mainly for implants	0, 1, 2, 3	0 = no visible plaque 1 = plaque recognised by running probe over smooth margin of implant 2 = visible plaque 3 = abundance of soft matter

of bleeding should be considered carefully due to the differences in the soft tissue interface between implants vs teeth with delayed bleeding indicating the possibility of trauma to the delicate soft tissue interface (Figure 7.5). Due to the orientation of the soft tissue, false positives can be elicited when probing around implants, and pressures of 0.15 N have been advocated. Thus, if the bleeding around an implant is a single dot then it is more likely to be related to tissue trauma; however, a continuous line of immediate

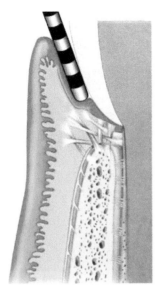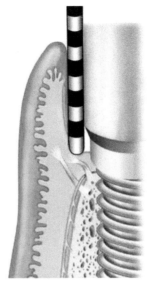

Figure 7.5 Showing the probing depths around teeth and implants and the resistance of the attachment to the probe penetration; the ability to probe along the long line axis of the implant will be dictated by the design and shape of the implant-retained crown or prosthesis (reproduced intechopen - I am asuming that perimissions have been sought).

bleeding is indicative of inflammation. Nevertheless, no bleeding on probing has a high negative predictive value indicating tissue stability. Bleeding around implants should be used in conjunction with other parameters such as the probing depth measurements. Suppuration may be detected around the sites, and although this is not a specific marker of peri-implant disease, its presence should be noted and monitored.

- Probing depths
  The use of probes around dental implants was controversial with challenges associated with the type of probe to use with plastic probes specifically designed for use around implants being advocated. However, it is now accepted that metal probes such as the UNC15, if used correctly, will not damage the implant surface or the soft tissue interface. Probing is now accepted as an important and reliable diagnostic tool in the longitudinal monitoring of the peri-implant tissues. The measurements should be recorded from the mesiobuccal running to the distobuccal and then from the mesiopalatal to the distopalatal using a reference point from which to measure the depth and a six point chart being recorded. The probing measurement should use a fixed reference point against which all future depths assessed. The access to the site for probing will also be dependent on the design and shape of the prosthesis and any challenges should be documented (Figure 7.6). The baseline probing depths should be recorded once the prosthesis is fitted and future recordings measured against this. Unlike teeth, there is no standard probing depth around implants due to the parallel nature of the long junctional epithelium resulting in the probing being down to bone as well as the different depths to which implants are placed. The depth of penetration of the probe will be dependent on the pressure used as well as the shape of the prosthesis and the connection to the implant (internal or external), the design of the system (one piece or two

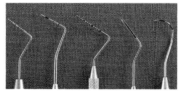

a. Range of probes (starting from left to right) William probe,
BPE probe, UNC15 probe, Flat probe, Nabers Furcation probe

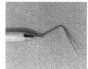

b. UNC15 probe

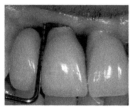
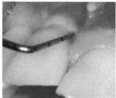

c. Probing around implants showing difficulty accessing
the mesial of the crown due to the contour

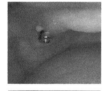

d.

Figure 7.6   a, b, c, d: Probing depth measurement using a UNC15 probe undertaken around an implant; The figure on the right (b) shows the difficulty of accessing the mesial of the crown due to the contour and c shows the use of a plastic probe around an implant with pus discharge.

piece) and the type/shape of the implant. The degree of recession around the implants should also be recorded as this will expose the implant threads leading to a higher risk of plaque accumulation (Figure 7.7a).

- Implant-retained prosthesis
  The prosthesis should be checked for the presence of plaque and its cleansability (Figure 7.8a, b, c, d). The mobility should be assessed either manually or using automated means such as the resonance frequency analyser (Ostell, Germany) or the Periotest. The cause of the mobility should be established and the reasons for the mobility assessed. Managing the mobility around single units is much easier than when noted around fixed multiunit linked restorations. These restorations should have been planned with retrievability and contingency in mind and if screw retained will be easier

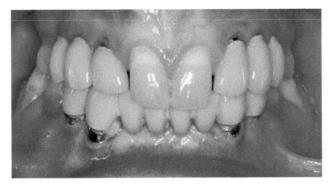

Figure 7.7a Recession around implants that have been in situ for > 10 years showing accumulation of calculus around the LR 3 implant. The thin quality of the gingival tissue biotype is evident but there are no probing depths as the patient has excellent plaque control.

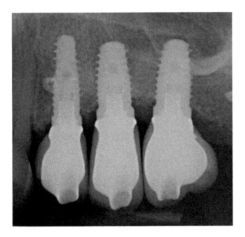

Figure 7.7b Bone levels around implants: they should remain stable after the initial remodelling that is seen during the first two years.

to remove and assess. Mobility can be at different levels and can be due to the prosthetic or abutment screw becoming loose or the implant becoming loose in which case it has failed (Figure 7.9a, b). Looseness of implants can be noted by palpating on the labial/buccal aspect of the implant and eliciting the mobility. The movement will be apparent along the long line axis whereas with a loose crown this will be limited to the area above the gingival margin. The occlusion should also be checked and any obvious wear faceting noted. Mobility, screw loosening and bone loss is related to unfavourable occlusal loading. Evidence of fracture of the veneering material should be noted and the cause established. Patients who have a grinding habit (parafunction) should be given a recommendation to wear a hard acrylic night guard to protect the implant-retained restorations and teeth. The hygienist/therapist during their assessment should be able to detect mobility and escalate the concerns if present to the dentist.

- Bone levels

  Radiographs should be taken normally following the fit of the prosthesis and then at 3, 6 and 12 months and annually for the first two years and then once every two years based on clinical need. This first year is critical due to the bone remodelling that takes place; however, many clinicians do not take radiographs at these timelines and only when there are concerns. The limitation of this approach is that if there is no baseline radiograph showing the bone levels, then future change in the bone levels will be difficult to establish. Radiographs should also be taken as adjuncts to the clinical assessment and not as part of a routine protocol and should have a sound clinical basis and rationale. The technique used should be standardised where possible with periapical radiographs being the most common. The change in the bone levels should be assessed against a marked reference point. The baseline radiographs taken after the fit of the restoration should be used to monitor the changes in the bone level and should take into account the post fit remodelling around the coronal part bearing in mind that the two-piece implant systems will show slightly more changes (1.5 mm during the first year followed by 0.1 mm annually thereafter) than the one-piece implant systems (Figure 7.7b). In recent years, attempts have been made to reduce the amount of bone remodelling seen marginally by the introduction of microthreading at the implant neck and platform switching by moving the microgap away from the gingival tissue interface. Thus, a knowledge of the different implant systems is important to help interpret the bone-level changes that may be seen. Hygienists/therapists should take note of the bone levels on radiographs that have been taken and assess these against the clinical assessments they undertake and interpret them accordingly.

At the end of the clinical assessment, a decision will be made as to whether the peri-implant tissues are healthy or whether there are any issues of concern. If the maintenance care is being undertaken by a hygienist/therapist, then they should ensure that concerns noted are escalated to the dentist so that appropriate measures can be implemented to manage the issue. In the event of a query from the patient or lack of clarity about the findings, a discussion should take place with the dentist and this could include information about the most appropriate maintenance regime for that patient. If the tissues are noted to be healthy, then the patient should be reminded of the importance of their daily cleaning and based on their risk profile, either a three-month or shorter-time interval follow-up appointment should be arranged.

During the first year the close monitoring of the peri-implant tissues is important and if the situation remains stable during this period, then the time intervals could be extended; however, the need for this should be balanced against the patients' ability to maintain the plaque control, the prosthetic design and their risk profile. Clinical signs of inflammation will indicate the presence of disease, and protocols outlined in the earlier chapter should be followed to manage the situation.

Intervals for Maintenance Care

The intervals considered will rely on the patients risk profile and risk predictors as well as the findings at each maintenance visit. The intervals should not be set in stone and should be customised according to the patients' needs and their risk profile which could change during the course of the monitoring. The risk profile is determined by the patients' age, ability to perform oral hygiene, medical risk factors, prosthetic risk factors and previous history of dental disease and biological/mechanical complications. There is limited evidence indicating the time intervals; however, clinical practice guidelines for healthy patients with implant retained restorations have been published by the American College of Prosthodontics and are based on a classification system that references the levels of published evidence (Table 7.2). They make the following recommendations:

- Patient Recall: Life long once every 6 months; higher risk patients need a more frequent assessment
- Professional Maintenance:
  Implant-Retained Removable Prosthesis (Overdentures and Partial)

Table 7.2 Clinical Practice Guidelines to Assess Peri-Implant Tissues and Recall Intervals (Bidra et al. 2016). Recommendations are categorised as A, B, C, D based on the strength of the published evidence shown on the left of the table.

Levels and Category of Evidence:

Ia: Systematic Review of Randomised Controlled Trials: *Graded A*

Ib: At least one Randomised Controlled Trial: *Graded A*

IIa: Once controlled study without randomisation: *B (extrapolated from Category I)*

IIb: One other type quasi-experimental study (time series analysis/studies where the unit of analysis is not the individual): *B (extrapolated from Category I)*

III: Non-experimental descriptive studies (comparative studies, cohort, case control): *Graded C (extrapolated from Category I or II evidence)*

IV: Expert committee reports, opinions or clinical experience of respected authorities: *Graded D (extrapolated from Category I, II, III)*

Topic	Guideline	Strength of Recommendation
1. Recall	• Assessment once every six months • High Risk: More frequently then six months depending on risk	D
2A. Professional Maintenance Removable Restorations – Dentures (Biological)	• Extra and Intraoral check; OHI for the implants and prosthesis; Intervention • Chlorhexidine should be used as an adjunct when needed clinically • Compatible cleaning instruments should be used including powered instruments including air polishers • Recommend appropriate topical agents	A, C, D
2B. Professional Maintenance Removable Restorations – Dentures (Mechanical)	• Detailed examination and patient education of possible future problems • Undertaken adjustment, repair, replacement or remake of prosthesis if needed	C, D

(Continued)

Table 7.2: (Continued)

Topic	Guideline	Strength of Recommendation
2 C. Professional Maintenance Fixed Restorations – Crowns, bridges (biological)	• Extra and Intraoral check; OHI for the implants and prosthesis; Intervention • Chlorhexidine should be used as an adjunct when needed clinically • Compatible cleaning instruments should be used including powered instruments including air polishers • Removal of the prosthesis will depend on patients ability to clean • Consider replacing the prosthetic screws if prosthesis is removed	A, C, D
2D. Professional Maintenance Fixed Restorations – Crowns, bridges (Mechanical)	• Detailed examination and patient education of possible future problems • Undertaken adjustment, repair, replacement or remake of prosthesis if needed • Consider new prosthetic screws when restoration is removed • Clinical signs indicate wear, then an occlusal splint should be made to protect the restorations including maintenance of the device; advised to wear at night • Oral topical agents should be recommended	C, D
3A. At Home Maintenance Removable	• Patient education about brushing the prosthesis and teeth using specified oral hygiene aides (floss, water flossers, interdental cleaners, brushing) • Cleaning at least twice daily around the teeth and implants • Prosthesis should be cleaned twice daily • Remove the prosthesis when sleeping and store in water or prescribed solution	C, D
3B. At Home Maintenance Fixed	• Patient education about brushing the prosthesis and teeth using specified oral hygiene aides (floss, water flossers, interdental cleaners, brushing) at least twice daily • Topical agents and intermittent use of chlorhexidine when needed • Wear the occlusal device at night if given one • Clean the device with soft brush and water and advice on care	A, C, D

a. Biological:
   Applies to issues with the tissues and the bone levels
   - Assessment as outlined earlier in conjunction with oral hygiene instructions for the implants and the prosthesis
   - Use of chlorhexidine gluconate as the oral topical agent
   - Professional scaling using hand and powered instrumentation compatible with the implants and prosthetic materials

- Professional cleaning of the prosthesis
- Appropriate oral hygiene aides and topical agents for use at home

b. Mechanical:

Applies to any issues with the prosthesis.
- Assessment of the prosthesis
- Perform adjustment or repair or give advice or remake parts of the prosthesis that have failed

Implant-Retained Fixed Prosthesis (single crowns, multiunit bridges and full reconstruction)

a. Biological:
- Assessment as outlined earlier
- Oral hygiene instructions for the implants and the prosthesis
- Use of chlorhexidine gluconate as the oral topical agent
- Professional scaling using hand and powered instrumentation compatible with the implants and prosthetic materials
- Removal of the prosthesis for professional cleaning will depend on patients' manual dexterity and the prosthetic contours modified for access if necessary (Figure 7.8a, b) with consideration being given to replacing the screws when reconnecting the prosthesis
- Appropriate oral hygiene aides and topical agents for use at home

b. Mechanical:
- Assessment of the prosthesis
- Repair, adjust or remake any parts that could impair function and aesthetics
- Consider new prosthetic screws especially in those who parafunction if the prosthesis is removed and replaced for professional mechanical maintenance
- Where there are marked wear facets or repeated issues with screw loosening, then consideration for a acrylic guard should be made for night-time wear with instruction on cleaning the device
- Remove loose cement-retained restorations and clean and recement (Figure 7.9a, b)
- Consider the use of adjuncts such as duraphat where there are still multiple teeth present

• Home Care:

Removable Prosthesis (Overdentures and Partial)
- Education about the use of manual and electric tooth brushes and the need to brush the natural teeth and the implant-retained prosthesis daily, removing the palque effectively and efficiently. Additional aides such as interdental cleaners, floss, and water picks (flossers) should be discussed.
- Sites around the implants should be cleaned effectively using soft brushes.
- Education about looking after the removable prosthesis should be given with the prosthesis being removed at night and the implants and prosthesis cleaned. The prosthesis should be stored in cold water or an appropriate cleaning solution.

Fixed Prosthesis (Single unit and Multiunit)

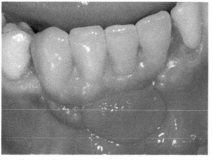 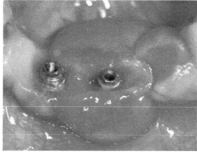

a, b: Flange of the prosthesis making cleaning difficult causing the tissue overgrowth; Extent of tissue swelling after removal of prosthesis

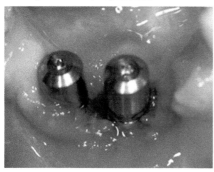 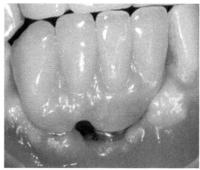

c, d: Excess tissue removed and prosthesis adjusted before refitting

Figure 7.8 a, b, c, d: Implant-retained prosthesis compromising the cleaning. The prosthesis was removed and the flange adjusted as part of the management.

- Education about the use of manual and electric tooth brushes and the need to brush the natural teeth and the implant-retained prosthesis daily removing the palque effectively and efficiently. Additional aides such as interdental cleaners, floss and water picks (flossers) should be discussed.
- Sites around the implants with multiple and complex reconstructions should be cleaned effectively using soft brushes and guidance given on the use of adjunctive topical chlorhexidine when necessary.
- Cleaning around the occlusal devices when recommended should be considered and the patient shown how to undertake this.

The time intervals for maintenance are predominantly based on case studies and limited data with six months being the most common interval. Patients with a history of periodontal disease and conditions such as oral mucosal disorders, bruxism, xerostomia and peri-implant disease would need to follow a similar protocol but will need additional support and may need to be seen more frequently. Patients who present during their maintenance period, with mechanical complications should be referred to the dentist for advice and guidance.

Treatment During a Maintenance Care Visit:

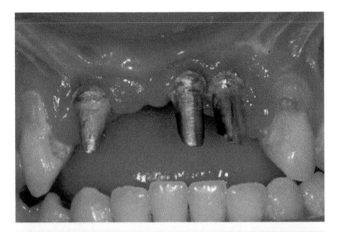

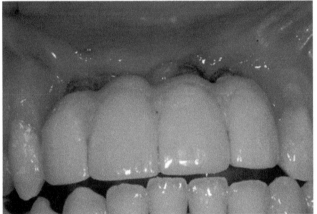

Figure 7.9 a, b: Loose cemented bridge showing abundant plaque on the abutments when the bridge was removed.

1. Patient education and reinforcement of the plaque control and home measures being used.

   Patient education will include double checking what the patient is using at home and reminding them of the need to keep up with effective daily cleaning, highlighting areas of concern, providing further guidance on choice of aides and frequency of use. Emphasis should be placed on reminding patients of the need to position electric/battery-operated brushes correctly with reference to the prosthesis and the gingival tissue margin. The interdental aides used for cleaning around implants are shown in Figure 7.10a–d. The way in which these aides are used is important to avoid and minimise the risk of trauma to the gingival tissues. The type of interdental brushes used should mirror the size of the embrasure spaces. The waterpick is a useful tool for flushing away soft plaque debris and should be recommended as an adjunct to normal cleaning. Patients should be warned about getting soaked when first starting to use it and advised to use it at least once daily before going to bed after the normal cleaning has been undertaken. The aide for cleaning

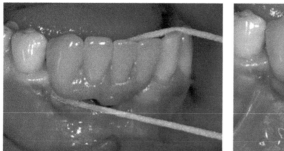
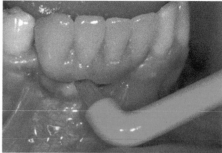

(a) Floss being used under the prosthesis

(b) Floss being used under the prosthesis

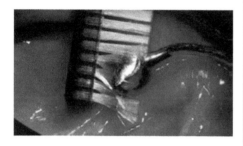
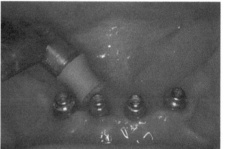

(c) Toothbrushing around the bar

(d) Rubber cup being used around locator abutments

Figure 7.10 a–d: Different oral hygiene aides that can be used for cleaning.

should be aligned with the patients' manual dexterity. The advice given should be in simple terms, concise and clear, such that the patient is not overburdened with information with many choices on multiple tools to use, as information overload is likely to lead to confusion and patient demotivation. The need to use positive and encouraging language is the door to a successful partnership with the patient and congratulating the patient when appropriate helps maintain their interest and engagement.

2. Instrumentation

The aim of the instrumentation during non-surgical therapy is to disrupt the biofilm and remove calculus.

Different types of instruments have been used for this and include the following: Scaling and root placing involves the use of currettes and fine polishing pastes to remove the soft and hard deposits. These old definitions have now become superseded by the term "professional mechanical plaque removal (PMPR)" which describes the professional mechanical removal of supragingival plaque and calculus with subgingival debridement to the depth of the sulcus/pocket. The terms supragingival PMPR and subgingival PMPR are the current terms used and are integral to the S3 clinical Practice Guidelines advocated for the management of periodontitis by the European Federation of Periodontology. These guidelines use a 3 stage approach with behavioural changes being an integral part of stage 1 along with risk factor management followed by the stage 2 and 3. These steps should be followed when managing peri-implant disease.

- Traditional ultrasonic tips should be used with caution as they can scratch the implant change; however, recent advances with plastic covered and coated tips have been shown to offer minimal effects on the surface. Polishing with fine polishing pastes using rubber cups and brushes has also been shown to have a positive effect on the outcome.
  - Hand instrumentation
    A number of different scalers have been used and include plastic, carbon fibre, titanium and gold tip currettes; however, each type can cause minor scratches on the abutment surface and thus should be used carefully. Whilst the plastic instruments seemingly cause the least damage, they also are the least effective at debridement due to the size and shape. In sites where the implant threads have been exposed, the use of titanium brushes has been advocated; however, the issues with small bristles being left behind have raised concerns about their use (Figure 7.11 a,b).
  - Machine-driven instrumentation
    Ultrasonic and sonic-driven devices have been used. Most manufacturers are now providing customised tips with plastic sleeves/inserts for cleaning around implants. These devices have been shown to provide the best cleaning effectiveness along with air powder abrasives. Whilst the latter has become popular in recent years, the efficacy of these remains open to question. Air polishing involves the use of glycine powders which are less abrasive than sodium bicarbonate with special inserts that allow the powder application and flushing. There are, however, reports indicating the risk of residual powder remaining in the site after treatment. Rotating rubber cups and brushes with prophylaxis paste have also been used, and it is noted that this may still cause some scratching and random pitting causing surface irregularities on the titanium (Figure 7.12).

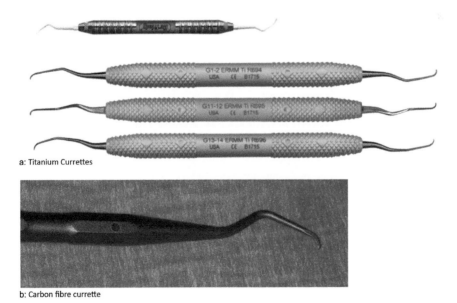

a: Titanium Currettes

b: Carbon fibre currette

Figure 7.11 a, b: Showing the different currettes used for scaling around implants.

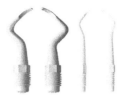

(a) Plastic curette inserts

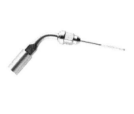
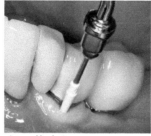

(b) Specialised insert used for debridement around implants

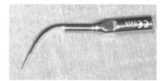

(c) Gold tipped insert for use with ultrasonic scalers

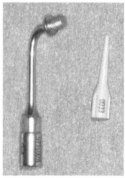
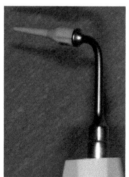
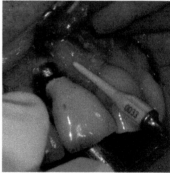

(d) Plastic insert that screws into the piezosurgery unit. Although shown for use with surgery, it can be used non surgically as well

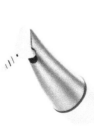
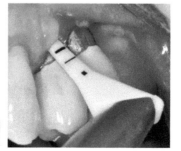

(e) Air flow Polisher

Figure 7.12   a, b, c, d, e: Showing the ultrasonic inserts and the airflow polisher.

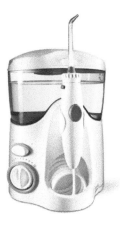

Figure 7.13   Water pick/flosser.

- Other treatment

  Patients where mechanical issues with the prosthesis are noted should be immediately referred to the dentist for management. The treatment protocols for sites with peri-implant disease have been covered in the previous chapter; however, those patients with advanced problems and non-responding sites should be discussed with the dentist.

  Water pick/flossers (Figure 7.13) are useful aides that help with flushing away the soft debries and are useful in patients with compromised manual dexterity.

Criteria for Success and Failure Dental Implant Retained Restorations

Chapter 2 covered the success and survival rates of dental implants. However, with newer implant designs and surface topography introduced by manufacturers, the success and survival data should be interpreted with caution as these cannot be directly extrapolated to the newer system designs. Currently, with the lack of any objective testing to determine implant success, surrogate outcome measures or treatment end points are used to measure success. These measures include probing depths, bleeding on probing and crestal bone loss along with pain and recession. As described earlier in this book, survival simply reflects the presence or absence of an implant irrespective of the health of the peri-implant tissues. Clinicians should be vigilant in monitoring the disease and supporting the hygienist/therapist in managing the patient with either ailing or failing implants ensuring that the patient has been made aware of the situation. The clinical criteria recommended by the Association of Dental Implantology to describe the state of the implants is shown in Table 7.3 and should be used during the monitoring phase.

Table 7.3 Definition of Implant Success and Failure (ADI Guidelines)

Success	Failing
Stable marginal bone levels after an initial crestal bone loss of <1.5mm	<50% progressive bone loss which has not stabilised
No BOP	BOP
PD <4mm	Deep pocketing
No mobility	Pain
Good plaque control (FMPI <20%)	Good plaque control (FMPI <20%)
	Exudate and discharge
At Risk	**Failed**
Initial bone loss of <4mm but bone loss has been stabilised	Discharge
PD <5mm	Deep pocketing
No BOP immediate or delayed	BOP
PI less than ideal	Mobility
	Lost or about to be lost

Key Learning Points

- Describe the importance of maintenance
- Discuss the components of maintenance
- Explain the steps to follow when issues are noted
- Consider the challenges in assessing tissues around implants and teeth
- Apply the criteria used for success around implant-retained restorations

References

1 Fody, A. (2020). Importance of Implant Maintenance. *Dimension of Dental Hygiene* 18 (4): 16–18, 21.
2 Bidra, A., Daubert, D., Garica, L., Kosinski, F. et al. (2016). Clinical Practice guidelines for recall and maintenance of patient with tooth borne and implant borne dental restorations. *Journal of American Dental Association* 147 (1).
3 Ucer, C., Scher, E., West, N., Retzepi, M., Simpson, S., Slade, K., and Donos, N. ADI guidelines on peri-implant monitoring and maintenance.
4 Drewenski, A.M. (2009). Hygiene and the implant patient: A preventive perspective. *RDH*.
5 Berglundh, T., Genco, R., Aass, A.M., Demirel, K., Derks, J., Figuero, E., Giovannoli, J.L., Goldstein, M., Lambert, F., Ortiz-Vigon, A., Polyzois, I., Salvi, G.E., Schwarz, F., Serino, G.,

Tomasi, C., and Zitzmann, N.U. (2015). Primary preention of peri-implantitis:managing peri-implant mucositis: Søren Jepsen[1]. *Journal of Clinical Periodontology* Suppl 16: 152–157.

6 Lin, C.Y., Chen, Z., Pan, W.L., and Wang, H.L. (2019). The effect of supportive **care** in preventing peri-**implant** diseases and **implant** loss: A systematic review and meta-analysis. *Clinical Oral Implants Research* 30 (8 Aug): 714–724.

7 Renvert, S., Hirooka, H., Polyzois, I., Kelekis-Cholakis, A., and Wang, H.L., and Working Group 3 (2019). Diagnosis and non-surgical treatment of peri-**implant** diseases and maintenance **care** of patients with dental **implants** – Consensus report of working group 3. *International Dental Journal* 69 (Suppl 2 Sep): 12–17.

8

Role of the Hygienist/Therapist

The successful outcome of dental implant treatment is dependent on team integration and team working. The members of this team are shown in Figure 8.1. The dental hygienist/therapist is an important member of this team and plays an essential and important role in the management of patients seeking implant treatment and the value of this role should not be underestimated. The involvement of the hygienist/therapist should not be an afterthought but should be considered right at the start of the treatment discussion. This position is further exemplified in patients who are at high risk of complications. To fulfil this role, training is important for the hygienist/therapist as part of the dental team and can be obtained through manufacturer-led programmes, private providers, hospitals and universities. Online training opportunities are also available, and the hygienist/therapist should take on the responsibility of ensuring that he/she is familiar with the management of patients with dental implants. Training, ideally, should be delivered through a team approach whereby the whole dental team, including the hygienist/therapist and the dentist, dental nurse and technician can learn together to appreciate the important role each member has in providing safe and optimal implant care to the patient. Training for hygienists and therapists in implantology is limited, and these team members must ensure that they are familiar with the concepts of different implant systems and treatment modalities to be able to provide effective treatment to the patients they see and escalate issues of concern in a timely manner.

As the field of implantology continues to evolve with different procedures, techniques, materials and products emerging onto the market, continuing education and lifelong learning is an important and essential part of the hygienist/therapists professional journey. As more and more patients are undergoing implant treatment, this need for awareness and knowledge has become even more critical especially as the extent to which this is taught at pre-registration level remains limited. The need for the ongoing learning is also driven by the high emotions and expectations patients hold around their implant restorations and the ability to impart clear and accurate information is reliant on sound knowledge and awareness. This chapter aims to provide an outline of the stages during which the hygienist/therapist will be involved in managing a patient who is undergoing or has undergone implant treatment.

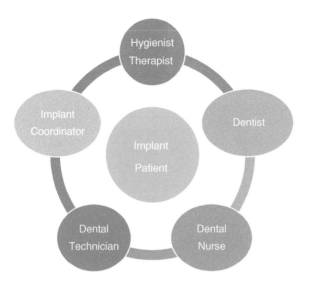

Figure 8.1 Members of the dental team involved in implant treatment.

Role as a Clinician

The role of the hygienist/therapist in caring for patients undergoing dental implant treatment can be broken down into the following stages (Figure 8.2):

- Before treatment – preoperatively
- During treatment
- After treatment – post-operatively

To be effective in their role, the hygienist/therapist should have an awareness and understanding of the key differences associated between the various implant systems and the types of implant-retained restorations provided to patients. There should be an insight into the nuances of treating teeth and dental implants and an awareness of the consequences of the treatment they may offer to a patient with an implant-retained reconstruction. He/she should also have the confidence of raising concerns when the signs of inflammation are noted. The current litigious climate, in which patients are highly aware of implant treatment through information gained from the internet, places the hygienist /therapist at a greater risk of medicolegal litigation. Thus, the need to have a good understanding of not only their role but also the self-awareness of their own limitations when providing treatment to patients who have undergone implant treatment should not be under-estimated.

- Before Treatment – Preoperatively

The hygienist/therapist plays an essential role during this phase in helping the patient understand their role in the management and success of their implant treatment. During this phase, the patient should be guided on how to optimise their day-to-day plaque control and the aides that should be used, shown and considered in line with the situation in the mouth. This will give the opportunity of determining aides that are easy for the patient to use and those that they would struggle with. In addition to this, if the patient is a smoker, then smoking cessation advice should be given and the importance of this highlighted to the patient alongside discussing other issues present around the teeth. Other preventative measures such as using fluoride mouthrinses should be implemented if necessary. In patients with gingivitis, treatment is undertaken to stabilise the disease. In patients with periodontitis, the hygienist/therapist has the dialogue with the patient about the importance of stabilising the disease before the implant treatment and explain the effects of the unstable disease on the outcome to the implant treatment. Patient engagement and the role they play in looking after their implants should be clarified at the outset and the patient advised of the poorer outcome to the implant treatment if they fail to comply. Challenges with patient compliance should be discussed with the dentist early so that the required modifications to the planned implant treatment made to ensure a successful result for the proposed treatment. This is an important part of the patient journey into implant treatment. At the end of this phase, a dialogue between the hygienist/therapist and dentist should take place outlining any major issues encountered and the outcome to the initial treatment. A record of the periodontal health and oral hygiene status should be kept and should include the plaque and bleeding scores as well as a six point probing chart. The patients progress and compliance to advice given should be assessed against this over the coming visits. Patients may also ask hygienist/therapists about their views on the proposed implant treatment and thus coherent and clear information can only be given if the hygienist/therapist has been part of the initial dialogue with the patient.

● During Treatment

The patient may be seen at various stages during this period. These are:

– Following the surgical placement of the implants
The hygenist/therapist may be asked to undertake the one-week post-surgery review. At this visit, guidance on how to change the cleaning regime in line with the surgical intervention is undertaken. Sutures should be removed and gentle cleaning with a soft brush and Corsodyl mouthrises should be advocated. The oral hygiene in the rest of the mouth assessed and the patient gently reminded that whilst brushing, the surgical site should be avoided, the rest of the mouth should be managed as normal. At this visit, any patient concerns are listened to, heard and escalated to the dentist if necessary.

– During the interim period whilst the implants are healing
The patient is given ongoing guidance and supportive care needed. If they had seen the patient prior to the start of the implant treatment, then the rapport built with the patient will help progress this phase whereby the hygienist can build on the information already given and monitor the patients performance against this. The hygienist/therapist will also be in a good position to identify untoward issues and escalate these if needed. Often they may see the patient just prior to the impression taking visit to ensure that the plaque control and gingival tissues around the implant sites are healthy so that an accurate impression can be obtained for the construction of the prosthesis.

– Following the fit of the prosthesis
This visit could be immediately after the fit or within days/weeks of the appointment. At this time, guidance on how to look after the implant-retained prosthesis will be given. For a removable prosthesis advice on how to clean the prosthesis should also be given and would include the following:

○ Remove and clean the prosthesis after every meal and rinse the mouth.

○ Leave the denture out at night and clean the denture and leave it soaked in cold water or a proprietary denture-cleaning solution.

○ Clean the denture with a brush and soap and water. Toothpaste is abrasive and can wear the material which the denture is made from.

○ The implant fixtures and abutments should be cleaned and all plaque and debris removed using either interspace brushes or a combination of aides. A waterpick will help with the removal of the soft debris.

For a fixed prosthesis the advice and guidance given will be dependent on the type of prosthesis which can be a single crown, bridge retained on a couple of implants or extensive full-arch reconstruction retained on the implant fixtures with either screws or cement. The postoperative care given should include the following:

○ Show the patient how to access the sites under the bridge and the aides to use to achieve this

○ Explain why the cleaning is of paramount importance

○ The toothbrushing and cleaning techniques should be revisited and customised to the needs of the patient and the type of prosthesis they have

○ The use of interspace, interproximal brushes and floss and waterpick should be advocated and checked

○ Excess cement that may be present should be removed

In both situations, a review visit within a few weeks should be arranged to ensure that the patient is able to perform the plaque-control measures discussed. Scaling and preventive advice is also undertaken if necessary.

● After Completion of Treatment

The hygienist/therapist will usually take the responsibility of the routine maintenance care of the patient. He/She should ask the patient if they have an 'implant passport' which will give them the required information about the implants. In the event this information is not available, then it should be requested from the treating dentist so that the correct maintenance plan can be executed. The hygienist/therapist should remember their duty of care and ensure that the information collected is documented and the clinical parameters collected are recorded and compared against the baseline assessment undertaken after the fit of the prosthesis. The steps outlined in the earlier chapter should be followed, data collected and recorded with measures implemented for patients who remain stable with healthy tissues and for those in whom signs of disease have been detected. The treatment intervention should align with the diagnosis of the condition and the treatment protocols outlined for the management of peri-implant mucositis and peri-implantitis in Chapter 6 should be followed. Any issues noted where the problem is beyond the scope of the hygienist/therapist should be discussed with the patient and a referral back to the dentist made so that the issues can be assessed, and early intervention sought. Patients with evidence of peri-implantitis should be discussed jointly with the dentist to ensure that the correct intervention plan is executed. The hygienist/therapist also has a responsibility to ensure that issues of concern are raised with the dentist timely so that treatment as needed can be initiated. The long-term monitoring of the implants will be vital and changes in medical conditions (e.g. uncontrolled diabetes) as well as recurrence of perio-dontitis in the periodontally susceptible patient with a history of periodontal disease should also be checked as these patients will be at a higher risk of disease progression. Smoking cessation should be an integral part of the management if smoking is an active issue. The long-term stability of the peri-implant tissues will be determined by meticulous plaque control and control of the occlusion both of which should be monitored more closely in the at-risk patient. Patients who have not been seen previously will start their journey slightly differently as the hygienist/therapist will need to implement the basic assessment and data collection outlined in the preoperative section and check the plaque control and initiate measures for treatment at this time. The rapport with the patient will take time to build with the hygienist/therapist driving the communication with the patient to ensure the best outcome is obtained. In these situations, the information about the patients implant treatment is even more crucial if the correct advice and guidance is to be given to the patient. The hygienist/therapist plays role as the early detector of peri-implant disease.

Role as an Educator

The hygienist/therapist has a substantial role as an educator in which they are responsible for imparting information to the patient about their plaque control and oral hygiene in language that is easy to understand for the patient who can then absorb and take on board the guidance given. In situations, where the patient's compliance remains consistently poor, the dentist should be alerted to this and the patient informed about the consequences of their noncompliance. The reasons for the rapid deterioration should be explained and the eventual failure and loss of the implant/s highlighted. The need for clear communica-tion is vital in this educator role and should be customised to meet with each patients needs and ability to grasp the information and assimilate it to help with their daily routine.

Figures 8.4a–e show the journey of a patient with periodontal disease with compro-mised upper anterior teeth that were extracted and replaced with an implant-retained reconstruction. The hygienist was integral to the provision of this treatment at the outset and went through the journey with the patient who became a highly motivated and com-pliant patient.

The main aspects of the implant treatment that the patient has undergone which the hygienist/therapist needs to be aware of are (Figure 8.3):

- The type of implant-related procedures that are being planned for the patient
- The actual procedure the patient has undergone
- The type of implant system used, i.e. one or two piece
- The type of surgical intervention that has taken place including information if soft tis-sue surgery and bone augmentation has been undertaken
- The type of prosthesis that has been provided including the type of retention, i.e. screw or cement retained
- The risk predictors and risk profile of the patient
- The instruments that should be used around implant-retained prosthesis

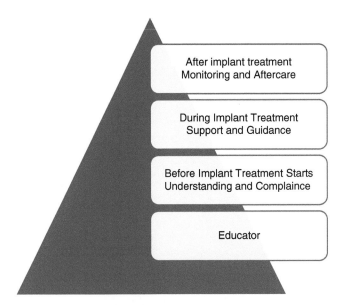

Figure 8.2 Role of the hygienist/therapist.

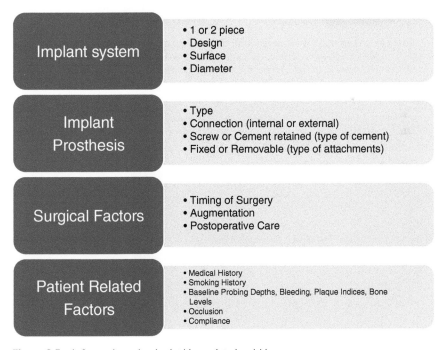

Figure 8.3 Information a hygienist/therapist should know.

This information should usually be provided to the patient at their end of their treatment by way of an 'implant treatment passport' and will help provide an overview of what needs to be done and the steps that need to be followed. The key systems information that the hygienist/therapist needs to be aware of is shown in Figure 8.2.

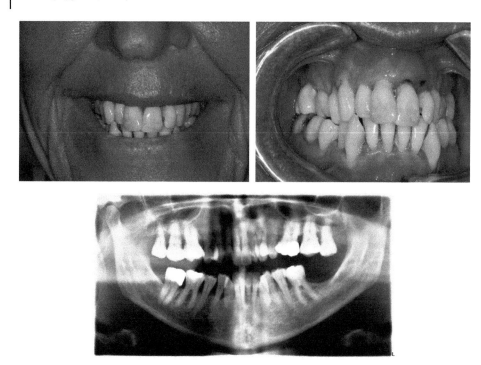

Fig 8.4a: Patient at presentation with periodontal disease and unhappy with the appearance of the upper anterior teeth which were failing. The preoperative radiograph shows calculus. The patient underwent treatment with the hygienist (before treatment).

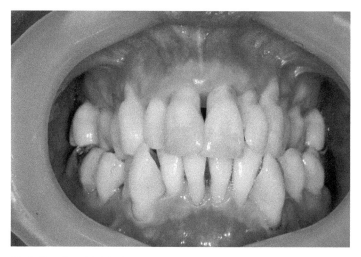

Fig 8.4b: Post initial phase therapy with the hygienist. The patient was educated in her role in managing her disease and the consequences of this if she was not able to optimise her cleaning. Note the healthy gingival tissues and she had no probing depths > 3–4 mm enabling the planning for the implant treatment to begin.

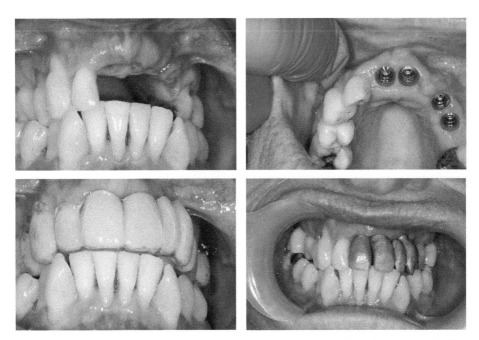

Fig 8.4 c: Patient following extraction of the upper anterior teeth with her interim prosthesis (Essix Retainer with teeth) and implant placement with the metal framework try in. She continued with treatment with the hygienist during this transitional phase.

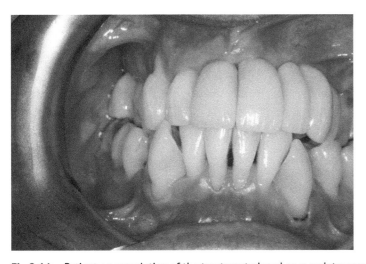

Fig 8.4d: Patient on completion of the treatment placed on a maintenance programme.

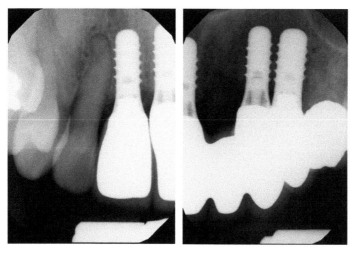

Fig 8.4e: Radiographs showing tissue level implants and the bone support.

Implant Systems

A knowledge and understanding of the implant systems is essential to help establish the correct type of maintenance treatment. It will also help the hygienist/therapist understand the precautions needed when providing the intervention and the instrumentation that should be used for treatment.

Implant Restoration Types

This helps ensure that the clinicians are able to deal with queries and questions the patient may ask with regards to knowing what to do. Additionally, an understanding of the materials used to construct the prosthesis will also help in choosing the correct instruments to use for the debridement. A knowledge of the systems used to connect the prosthesis to the implants is also important as patients may attend for their maintenance care with issues surrounding the prosthesis and this will help establish the need for referral. Additionally, the patient may ask for advice or the hygienist may notice movement of the crown or prosthesis and should be well informed to provide a response.

Surgical Procedures

If during maintenance a patient presents with problems around the implants with bone loss, then having the knowledge about the surgical options and the possible risks would empower the hygienist/therapist in sign posting the patient at the same as advising the

Table 8.1 Clinical Criteria Used to Describe Success and Failure around Implants (Association of Dental Implantology)

Success	Failing Implants
• Stable marginal bone levels after an initial crestal bone loss of < 1.5 mm (for two-piece systems) • No bleeding on probing • Probing depths < 4 mm • No mobility • Good plaque control (full-mouth plaque scores < 20%)	• 50% progressive bone loss which has not stabilised • Deep pocketing • Bleeding on probing • Pain • Exudate/discharge • Less than ideal plaque control
At Risk	**Failed**
• Initial bone loss of < 4 mm but bone loss has been stabilised • Probing depths < 5 mm • No bleeding on probing (immediate or delayed) • Plaque index is less than ideal	• Deep pocketing • Discharge • Bleeding on probing • Mobility • Lost or about to be lost

patient of the importance of seeking advice from a dentist as soon as possible. An understanding of the surgical procedures the patient has undergone for the implant placement also provides the hygienist/therapist a better understanding of the possible ways in which the maintenance care regime may need to be altered.

Table 8.1 shows the clinical criteria that can be used to describe success or failure around implants. These guidelines and steps should empower the hygienist/therapist to ensure that their position is established within the team providing care to an implant patient. The rapidly evolving and changing concepts along with advances in technology highlight the need for ongoing continuing professional development if patient care is to be delivered optimally. The development of a close, open and integrated working relationship with the treating dentist is essential as implant treatment for a patient cannot be seen as a one-off treatment but a lifelong journey during which turbulence with complications can be encountered at any stage which will need timely intervention. The hygienist/therapist by forearming themselves with the required information and knowledge will place themselves in a strong autonomous position in supporting and managing patients with implant treatment.

Key Learning Points

- Explain the role of the hygienist/therapist as a team member
- Discuss the stages at which the hygienist/therapist is involved
- Describe the components of the care that needs to be provided
- Appreciate the need for continuing professional development and ongoing learning

References

1 Fody, A. (2020). Importance of Implant Maintenance. *Dimension of Dental Hygiene* 18 (4 April): 16–18, 21.

2 Bidra, A., Daubert, D., Garica, L., Kosinski, F. et al. (2016). Clinical Practice guidelines for recall and maintenance of patient with tooth borne and implant borne dental restorations. *Journal of American Dental Association* 147 (1).

3 Ucer, C., Scher, E., West, N., Retzepi, M., Simpson, S., Slade, K., and Donos, N. ADI guidelines on peri-implant monitoring and maintenance.

4 Drewenski, A.M. (2009). Hygiene and the implant patient: A preventive perspective. *RDH*.

5 Berglundh, T., Genco, R., Aass, A.M., Demirel, K., Derks, J., Figuero, E., Giovannoli, J.L., Goldstein, M., Lambert, F., Ortiz-Vigon, A., Polyzois, I., Salvi, G.E., Schwarz, F., Serino, G., Tomasi, C., and Zitzmann, N.U. (2015). Primary preention of peri-implantitis:managing peri-implant mucositis: Søren Jepsen[1]. *Journal of Clinical Periodontology* Suppl 16: 152–157.

6 Lin, C.Y., Chen, Z., Pan, W.L., and Wang, H.L. (2019). The effect of supportive **care** in preventing peri-**implant** diseases and **implant** loss: A systematic review and meta-analysis. *Clinical Oral Implants Research* 30 (8 Aug): 714–724.

7 Renvert, S., Hirooka, H., Polyzois, I., Kelekis-Cholakis, A., and Wang, H.L., and Working Group 3 (2019). Diagnosis and non-surgical treatment of peri-**implant** diseases and maintenance **care** of patients with dental **implants** - Consensus report of working group 3. *International Dental Journal* 69 (Suppl 2 Sep): 12–17.

Index

Note: Page numbers in *Italics* refer to figures: those in **Bold** refer to tables.

Dental Implants for Hygienists and Therapists, First Edition. Ulpee Darbar.
© 2022 John Wiley & Sons Ltd. Published 2022 by John Wiley & Sons Ltd.